Managing the Complications of Cirrhosis

A Practical Approach

Managing the Complications of Cirrhosis

A Practical Approach

Edited by

Atif Zaman, MD, MPH
Professor of Medicine
Section Chief, Division of Gastroenterology and Hepatology
Director of Clinical Hepatology
Oregon Health & Science University
Portland, Oregon

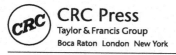

CRC Press
Taylor & Francis Group
Boca Raton London New York

CRC Press is an imprint of the
Taylor & Francis Group, an **informa** business

First published 2012 by SLACK Incorporated

Published 2024 by CRC Press
2385 NW Executive Center Drive, Suite 320, Boca Raton FL 33431

and by CRC Press
4 Park Square, Milton Park, Abingdon, Oxon, OX14 4RN

CRC Press is an imprint of Taylor & Francis Group, LLC

© 2012 Taylor & Francis Group, LLC

Library of Congress Cataloging-in-Publication Data

Managing the complications of cirrhosis : a practical approach / edited by Atif Zaman.
     p. ; cm.
  Includes bibliographical references and index.
  ISBN 9781556429576 (alk. paper)
  I. Zaman, Atif.
  [DNLM: 1. Liver Cirrhosis--complications. 2. Liver Diseases--therapy. WI 725]
  LC classification not assigned
  616.3'624--dc23
                         2011033813

ISBN: 9781556429576 (pbk)
ISBN: 9781003524977 (ebk)

DOI: 10.1201/9781003524977

DEDICATION

I would like to thank first and foremost my family: Doreen, my wife, who inspires me to be a better person every day; and my children, Kalyn and Evelyn, who are the true joys of my life. I would also like to thank all the patients who I have seen over the years; I have learned so much from them…and they have inspired this book.

Contents

ACKNOWLEDGMENTS

I would like to thank all of my colleagues, many of whom are authors in this book, for their friendship, camaraderie, advice, and mentorship.

In addition, we the authors would like to acknowledge our patients from whom we are constantly learning. In taking care of our patients we are privileged to witness the strength and perseverance of the human spirit.

Finally, I would like to thank SLACK Incorporated for their patience, support, and hard work, specifically Carrie Kotlar, Senior Acquisitions Editor; April Billick, Managing Editor; and Alanna Franchetti, Assistant Project Editor.

ABOUT THE EDITOR

Atif Zaman, MD, MPH, received his BS in Biomedical Engineering from Boston University in 1987, his MD from Tufts University, and his MPH from Oregon Health and Science University (OHSU) in 2000. He is currently Professor of Medicine in the Division of Gastroenterology and Hepatology and in the Department of Public Health and Preventive Medicine at OHSU. He is the Section Chief of the Division of Gastroenterology and Hepatology and the Director of Clinical Hepatology at OHSU.

Dr. Zaman's research has involved collaborations with a number of scientists and a series of clinical research projects. He is the Principal Investigator on numerous grants and is the recipient of the WAFMR Outstanding Investigator Award.

Dr. Zaman is a member of several national societies: the American Gastroenterological Association, the American College of Physicians, and the American Association for the Study of Liver Diseases. He has authored more than 50 manuscripts, review articles, and abstracts.

CONTRIBUTING AUTHORS

James R. Burton Jr, MD (Chapter 10)
Associate Professor of Medicine
Director of Liver Transplantation
Division of Gastroenterology and Hepatology
University of Colorado Hospital
Aurora, Colorado

Michael F. Chang, MD, MSc (Chapter 8)
Assistant Professor of Medicine
Department of Medicine
Division of Gastroenterology and Hepatology
Oregon Health & Science University
Portland Veterans Administration Medical Center
Portland, Oregon

Jonathan M. Fenkel, MD (Chapter 5)
Assistant Professor of Medicine
Jefferson Medical College
Division of Gastroenterology and Hepatology
Thomas Jefferson University Hospital
Philadelphia, Pennsylvania

Edoardo G. Giannini, MD, PhD, FACG (Chapter 4)
Assistant Professor
Gastroenterology Unit
Department of Internal Medicine
University of Genoa
Genoa, Italy

Kenneth Ingram, PA-C (Chapter 9)
Assistant Professor of Medicine
Division of Gastroenterology and Hepatology
Oregon Health & Science University
Portland, Oregon

Willscott E. Naugler, MD (Chapter 2)
Assistant Professor of Medicine
Department of Medicine
Division of Gastroenterology and Hepatology
Oregon Health & Science University
Portland, Oregon

Victor J. Navarro, MD (Chapter 5)
Division of Gastroenterology and Hepatology
Thomas Jefferson University Hospital
Philadelphia, Pennsylvania

Anna Sasaki, MD, PhD (Chapter 3)
Associate Professor of Medicine
Division of Gastroenterology and Hepatology
Veterans Administration Medical Center
Portland, Oregon

Jonathan M. Schwartz, MD (Chapter 7)
Associate Professor
Department of Medicine
Division of Gastroenterology and Hepatology
Oregon Health & Science University
Portland, Oregon

Jayant A. Talwalkar, MD, MPH (Chapter 6)
Associate Professor of Medicine
Division of Gastroenterology and Hepatology
Mayo Clinic
Rochester, Minnesota

PREFACE

Who needs this book?

This particular pocket textbook is geared toward the busy practitioner who sometimes sees patients with liver disease. It is essentially the management of cirrhosis for the nonhepatologist including general gastroenterologists, primary care practitioners, nurse practitioners/physician's assistants, hospitalists, and trainees. Each chapter highlights how to manage cirrhosis-related problems using simple tables and algorithms based on the current best evidence. Each chapter also provides complex cases where there is no standard treatment but there are emerging data. In future editions, these emerging data and issues will be specifically updated.

But why does a practitioner need such a book? The truth is that all practitioners will see an increasing number of patients with liver disease. Right now it is estimated that 5.5 million individuals have cirrhosis nationwide; over a 10-year period the rates of cirrhosis may increase by 61%.[1] With the rise of obesity, the rates of nonalcoholic fatty liver has increased and over time fatty liver disease can progress to cirrhosis. Furthermore, recent studies suggest that although the rate of new hepatitis C infection is not increasing, the rate of end-stage liver disease due to hepatitis C infection is rising as patients are chronically infected for longer and longer periods of time.[2]

Recent modeling studies suggest that over a 10-year period, the rates of cirrhosis may increase by 61%, liver-related complications by 279%, and liver-related death by 223%.[3,4] It should not surprise clinicians that patients presenting with cirrhosis and its complications—whether from hepatitis C infection, alcoholism, etc—will be more and more commonly seen. Therefore, practicing clinicians need to be well prepared to manage patients with cirrhosis, specifically its major complications.

REFERENCES

1. Kim WR, Brown RS, Terrault NA, El-Serag H. Burden of liver disease in the United States: summary of a workshop. *Hepatology.* 2002;36:227-242.
2. Deuffic-Burban S, Poynard T, Sulkowski MS, Wong JB. Estimating the future health burden of chronic hepatitis C and human immunodeficiency virus infections in the United States. *J Viral Hepat.* 2007;14:107-115.
3. Davis GL, Albright JE, Cook SF, Rosenberg DM. Projecting future complications of chronic hepatitis C in the United States. *Liver Transpl.* 2003;9:331-338.
4. Kim WR. The burden of hepatitis C in the United States. *Hepatology.* 2002;36(5 Suppl 1):S30-S34.

INTRODUCTION

Atif Zaman, MD, MPH

Cirrhosis is the end-stage consequence of fibrosis of the hepatic parenchyma. Once cirrhosis develops, progressive architectural distortion, nodule formation, and altered hepatic function are the hallmarks. The pathophysiology of hepatic fibrosis and ultimately cirrhosis has been recently clarified. The hepatic stellate cell (previously called the Ito cell) is the primary source of the extracellular matrix, the building blocks of fibrosis, in both the normal and fibrotic liver. These cells represent 15% of the cell population in the liver.[1] Stellate cell activation is considered the central event in hepatic fibrosis and its main stimuli is derived from hepatocyte injury. Thus, fibrosis of the liver develops as a result of a sustained wound-healing response to chronic liver injury from a variety of causes, including alcohol, hepatitis C infection, hepatitis B infection, hemochromatosis, and autoimmune diseases of the liver.

Clinically, cirrhosis can be diagnosed by one of 3 methods. First, histological examination of liver tissue—obtained via a percutaneous, transjugular, or surgical approach—allows the microscopic identification of cirrhosis. Second, imaging of the liver can identify gross distortions such as a shrunken nodular liver. Furthermore, abdominal imaging can identify portal hypertensive changes such as portal vein dilation, splenomegaly, ascites, and intra-abdominal varices. Finally, laboratory abnormalities can help identify cirrhosis. Thrombocytopenia in a patient with chronic liver disease is a reflection of splenomegaly related to portal hypertension and is highly suspicious of cirrhosis. Other laboratory evidence of cirrhosis includes elevated serum total bilirubin (which reflects

Zaman A. *Managing the Complications
of Cirrhosis: A Practical Approach* (pp 1-4).
© 2012 Taylor & Francis Group.

hepatic clearance dysfunction) and low serum albumin and elevated international normalized ratio (INR; which reflect hepatic synthetic dysfunction). In addition, physical exam findings such as palmar erythema, spider angiomas, ascites, asterixas, and caput medusa can be helpful, although they are not always present.

Therefore, if there is physical, laboratory, and/or radiologic evidence of cirrhosis, a liver biopsy is not necessary to verify the diagnosis.

PORTAL HYPERTENSION

Cirrhosis ultimately leads to a rise in portal pressure, the opening of porto-systemic collaterals, and systemic hemodynamic abnormalities that can ultimately affect other organs including the kidneys and lungs. This constellation of abnormalities is coined *portal hypertension syndrome.* Keep in mind that essentially all chronic liver diseases go through initial chronic injury that leads to fibrosis, followed by cirrhosis, and finally leads to portal hypertension syndrome. This syndrome can be described in 3 steps:

1. As hepatic fibrosis increases, there is increased distortion of the intrahepatic vasculature due to scar tissue. Furthermore, as a result of these anatomical changes, the balance between pro- and anticontractile elements is altered, favoring constriction. The increase in endothelin-1 production in stellate cells, the decrease in hepatic production of nitric oxide, and the increase in angiotensin and alpha-adrenergic stimulation all favor a contractile state in the liver.[2,3] This leads to an increase in intrahepatic resistance.

2. This increased intrahepatic resistance leads to an increase in the portal pressure. A portal pressure gradient between 10 and 12 mm Hg promotes the development of esophageal varices[4] and portal-systemic collaterals. Collateral development is due not only to the passive opening of closed vessels or redirection of flow in the splanchnic vascular bed but also to angiogenesis.[5] These anatomical alterations lead to esophagogastric varices, portal hypertensive gastropathy, and colopathy.

3. The above changes promote alterations in several other organs, leading to the full expression of portal hypertension syndrome. This includes the development of a hyperdynamic systemic circulation characterized by a decrease in systemic vascular resistance and a rise in cardiac output with a lower mean arterial pressure. Systemic vasodilation will result in relative arterial underfilling, which stimulates baroreceptors and volume receptors. This leads to the activation of the renin-angiotensin system and vasopressin release. Progressive arterial vasodilation causes renal arterial vasoconstriction with deleterious effects to the renal system, including the development of hepatorenal syndrome. Also, pulmonary

arterial vasodilation and shunting can lead to hepatopulmonary syndrome. Finally, portosystemic shunting leads to the escape of neurotoxins from the hepatic system into the systemic circulation. Once these neurotoxins reach the brain, a cascade of neurochemical alterations occur that can cause hepatic encephalopathy.

The development of portal hypertention syndrome leads to numerous complications of cirrhosis, including variceal hemorrhage, ascites, encephalopathy, and hepatorenal and hepatopulmonary syndromes. Because not every practicing clinician can subspecialize in hepatology, this book provides a management tool for these common conditions related to portal hypertension and cirrhosis. You will be seeing more of these complications, so be prepared.

REFERENCES

1. Geerts A. History, heterogeneity, developmental biology, and functions of quiescent hepatic stellate cells. *Semin Liver Dis.* 2001;21:311-335.
2. Iredale JP. Cirrhosis: new research provides a basis for rational and targeted treatments. *BMJ.* 2003;327:143-147.
3. Rockey DC. Vascular mediators in the injured liver. *Hepatology.* 2003;37:4-12.
4. Garcia-Tsao G, Groszmann RJ, Fisher RL, et al. Portal pressure, presence of gastroesophageal varices and variceal bleeding. *Hepatology.* 1985;5:419-424.
5. Lee FY, Colombato LA, Albillos A, et al. Administration of N omega-nitro-L-arginine ameliorates porto-systemic shunting in portal hypertensive rates. *Gastroenterology.* 1993;105:1464-1470.

PREVENTATIVE HEALTH ISSUES IN PATIENTS WITH CIRRHOSIS

Willscott E. Naugler, MD

Patients with cirrhosis may present for medical attention in various ways, from an asymptomatic patient in whom the diagnosis is made based on blood tests, imaging, etc, to the patient presenting with one or more of the major complications (eg, encephalopathy, ascites, variceal bleeding, or hepatocellular carcinoma [HCC]). In the last case, management of the complication (see relevant sections outlining management of complications) takes precedence over any preventative care. Once major complications have been addressed or if the patient has presented with compensated cirrhosis, attention may be directed toward identifying the possible development of complications that may be either prevented or minimized. For practical purposes, complications of cirrhosis whose natural history may be meaningfully altered include the development of variceal bleeding, HCC, and, to a lesser extent, osteoporosis. This chapter will focus on identification and preventative measures that apply to these 3 complications of cirrhosis.

HEPATOCELLULAR CARCINOMA

Epidemiology

HCC is a devastating cancer, with an incidence rate nearly identical to the annual mortality rate, indicating that most patients with HCC die within 1 year of diagnosis. In fact, HCC is the leading cause of death in patients with compensated cirrhosis, responsible for 54% to 70% of deaths in this group.[1,2] HCC is the third leading cause of cancer-related death worldwide,[3] and its

Zaman A. *Managing the Complications of Cirrhosis: A Practical Approach* (pp 5-18).
© 2012 Taylor & Francis Group.

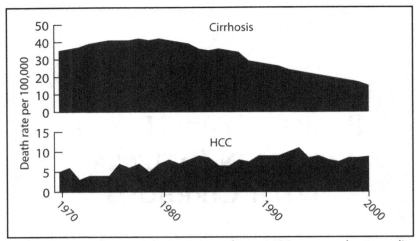

Figure 2-1. Mortality in cirrhotic patients due to HCC compared to mortality due to complications of cirrhosis. (Adapted from Fattovich G, Stroffolini T, Zagni I, Donato F. Hepatocellular carcinoma in cirrhosis: incidence and risk factors. *Gastroenterology.* 2004;127:S35-S50.)

incidence is rising in the United States[4] and other parts of the world.[5,6] Even more compelling are data showing that mortality due to complications of cirrhosis (other than HCC) is decreasing, whereas the rate of HCC-related mortality is rising (Figure 2-1).[7] These data suggest that management of non-HCC complications of cirrhosis (variceal bleeding, spontaneous bacterial peritonitis, etc) has been improving, allowing patients with cirrhosis to live longer and therefore be at increased risk of developing HCC.

Until better serum markers or molecular indicators of HCC are available, however, the field will rely on clinically known risk factors for the development of HCC. There are several identifiable etiologies that may lead to the development of HCC, the most common of which is infection with hepatitis B virus (HBV). **In areas of the world where HBV infection is endemic, it is the most common reason for the development of HCC and, indeed, the bulk of HCC worldwide stems from HBV infection.**[8] There is a striking similarity between world maps of HBV prevalence and HCC incidence. To highlight the importance of HBV infection as an etiology behind hepatocarcinogenesis, mass vaccination strategies were employed in Taiwan, resulting in a significant drop in new cases of HCC.[9] Similar strategies have been employed in other countries with similar success.[10,11]

Like HBV, hepatitis C virus (HCV) infection invites hepatocarcinogenesis. **Unlike HBV, however, HCV infection usually does not result in the development of HCC until after cirrhosis has occurred.** Fifteen percent to 35% of patients with HCV infection develop cirrhosis after 25 to 30 years.[12]

Good estimates put the incidence of hepatocarcinogenesis at 1% to 3% after 30 years of HCV infection.[13] HCC rarely occurs in the noncirrhotic liver with HCV infection, but once cirrhosis is established, primary liver cancer evolves at a rate of 1% to 3% per year.

Other clear risk factors for HCC development include alcohol use, hemochromatosis,[14] and nonalcoholic fatty liver disease (NAFLD).[15,16] Assessment of each of these risk factors has been somewhat problematic. In the case of alcohol use, most of the studies showing an increased risk of HCC were performed in the era prior to our ability to detect simultaneous HCV infection. Selected groups have shown that HCC develops at a rate of about 1% per year in the decompensated cirrhotic due to alcohol[17] and that drinking 80 g/day of alcohol over 10 years increases the risk of HCC 5-fold compared to nondrinking controls.

NAFLD and its more aggressive variant nonalcoholic steatohepatitis (NASH) are known to cause cirrhosis, and increasing data are implicating them in HCC development. As in other conditions that lead to cirrhosis, NASH is complicated by HCC usually in the context of advanced fibrosis or cirrhosis.[18] NAFLD itself often arises in the milieu of metabolic syndrome, defined by insulin resistance, hyperlipidemia, hypertension, and truncal obesity. Diabetes mellitus[15] and obesity[16,19] have themselves been implicated as risk factors for hepatocarcinogenesis, most likely through their association with NAFLD and its hepatic consequences.

It is generally accepted that most HCC (90% or more) develops in the background of advanced fibrosis or cirrhosis, with the notable exception of HBV infection. Thus, clinical risk factors for the development of primary liver cancer can be simply boiled down to these 2 groups: those with cirrhosis and those with HBV infection. Figure 2-2 details patients who should be screened for HCC and subsequently entered into a long-term HCC surveillance program.

Hepatocellular Carcinoma Screening and Surveillance

Screening and surveillance for HCC development in at-risk populations has become commonplace, but it is worthwhile to briefly address the rationale for this practice. *Screening* is the application of a test for the diagnosis of a problem in the absence of symptoms or another reason to suggest that the problem exists, and *surveillance* is the repeated application of such a test. For the purposes of HCC, this means the use of validated tests (scans and/or serum biomarkers) in at-risk populations (HBV infection and cirrhosis) at regular intervals over time. The ultimate goal, of course, is to detect HCC at a stage at which life-prolonging therapy is available, tolerable by the patient, and, ideally, cost-effective to society at large. These goals have guided current recommendations by the major hepatology societies.[20]

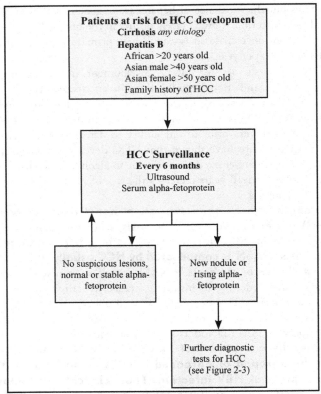

Figure 2-2. HCC screening/surveillance algorithm. (Based on the American Association for the Study of Liver Diseases recommendations found in Calle EE, Rodriguez C, Walker-Thurmond K, Thun MJ. Overweight, obesity, and mortality from cancer in a prospectively studied cohort of US adults. *N Engl J Med.* 2003;348:1625-1638.)

The management of HCC is complex and reviewed elsewhere in this book. Despite regional differences in treatment patterns, however, **a general rule concerning HCC is that treatment is largely determined by the amount of remaining hepatic reserve.** For patients with the most severe liver disease (Child's C cirrhotics), there is currently no therapy for HCC that will prolong survival, and indeed most treatments might hasten the demise of these patients. Such patients are at higher risk of dying from liver failure than from progression of HCC. Thus, screening patients with Child's C cirrhosis is not recommended because there are no HCC treatment options in this group. The exceptions are patients who are liver transplant candidates or listed for liver transplant. Screening for HCC in this group is reasonable with the rationale that transplant is a potentially curative treatment for HCC provided that it is within certain criteria,[21] and beyond these criteria a transplant is potentially futile due to high posttransplant recurrence rates.

Survival of patients diagnosed with symptomatic HCC is dismal, with 5-year survival rates of less than 10%. On the other hand, when HCC is discovered at an early stage such that resection or transplantation is possible, survival rates of 50% to 75% are now possible.[22,23] Even more exciting are studies showing that nonsurgical therapies (such as local radio-frequency ablation) may be able to achieve survival rates comparable to surgical resection.[24] Such good outcomes for this potentially devastating cancer are only achievable when it is caught at an early stage.

It should be acknowledged, however, that good outcomes depend not only on early detection through surveillance of at-risk populations but the availability of expertise in the treatment of HCC. The management of this cancer is complicated and rapidly evolving and includes hepatologists, surgeons, radiologists, interventional radiologists, radiation oncologists, and oncologists. Ideally, there is a team of such practitioners working in concert to care for the patient with HCC. And because liver transplant is one therapeutic (potentially curative) option, having such a multidisciplinary HCC treatment group at a liver transplant center is ideal. Thus, for the practitioner who identifies a patient at risk for the development of HCC, it is important to identify a center for HCC treatment prior to placing the patient in a surveillance program.

Once the at-risk patient has been identified, an evaluation has been made regarding whether the patient can tolerate treatment of HCC should it be determined, and a center for HCC treatment has been ascertained, the patient can be enrolled in an HCC screening and surveillance program. Currently available screening tools include serum biomarkers and various scans. Alphafetoprotein (AFP) is the most commonly used serum biomarker and there is a good deal of data detailing its operating characteristics. Unfortunately, the serum AFP has proven to be a poor screening test, with low positive predictive values no matter where the cutoff level is set. In a systematic analysis of 5 studies looking at the test characteristics of AFP, it had a sensitivity for HCC diagnosis of 41% to 65% and a specificity of 80% to 94% at a cutoff of 20 mcg/L.[25] As the AFP cutoff (for diagnosis of HCC) rises, the sensitivity decreases, whereas the specificity increases. As an example, with an AFP cutoff of 200 mcg/L, the sensitivity was found to be 22%, with 99% specificity. Nonetheless, a high AFP (>200 mcg/L) as well as a persistently high AFP have been found to be significant risk factors for HCC, and thus this test is a useful adjunct to scanning the patient at risk for HCC.

Other serum biomarkers have been developed, including, most notably, the des-gamma-carboxy prothrombin (DGCP), also known as prothrombin induced by vitamin K absence II (PIVKA II). Studies have been unable to show that it performs any better than the AFP alone, however. Still more markers have been investigated, and it is possible that in the near future some combination of these biomarkers will be able to more accurately discover early HCC. For the time being, however, AFP is the currently recommended biomarker but still only as an adjunct to the more accurate information gained from imaging.

Worldwide the most common imaging technique used for HCC screening is ultrasonography (US). A systematic review comparing US with computed tomography (CT) and magnetic resonance imaging (MRI) showed that US had a sensitivity of 60% and a specificity of 97% for the detection of HCC when compared to the gold standard of pathological examination.[26] Using a strategy of US every 6 months for HCC surveillance would result in a cost of about $2000 per tumor discovered. Because the sensitivity of US (with or without AFP) for HCC surveillance is not optimal, many practitioners in the United States alternate scanning the patient with US and another modality such as contrast-enhanced CT or MRI. There are no data to support this practice, however, and aside from increased cost with such a strategy, there are increasing concerns of the long-term effects (other cancers) caused by radiation exposure from multiple CT scans. In addition, tests used for the confirmation of HCC are generally not employed as screening tests. Given the complexity of making the diagnosis of HCC and the reliance on imaging, it is clear that collaboration with an experienced radiologist who is on the lookout for HCC will increase the chances of making this important diagnosis.

In patients at risk for HCC, recommended surveillance intervals are every 6 to 12 months. This recommendation is based on tumor doubling time, not the particular risk of the patient. Though there are no clear data to support the 6-month versus 12-month interval, studies showing a survival benefit from HCC surveillance used the 6-month interval, and most experts use the 6-month interval.[20] An algorithm for the screening and surveillance of HCC is outlined in Figure 2-2.

Diagnosis of Hepatocellular Carcinoma

When an at-risk patient has been entered into an HCC surveillance program and one of the surveillance tests suggest the development of cancer (new nodule on US and/or rising AFP), a confirmatory test or tests are usually necessary to establish the diagnosis. Because there is a small chance of tumor seeding with biopsy and given that there is a higher complication rate from biopsies in cirrhotic patients, noninvasive criteria for the diagnosis of HCC have been formed and validated.[20] Figure 2-3 outlines an accepted algorithm for the diagnosis of HCC. When the diagnosis of HCC has been secured, the patient should be referred to a multidisciplinary group familiar with the treatment of HCC (outlined in Bruix and Sherman[20]). **If confirmatory testing fails to make the diagnosis, patients can either revert to routine (every**

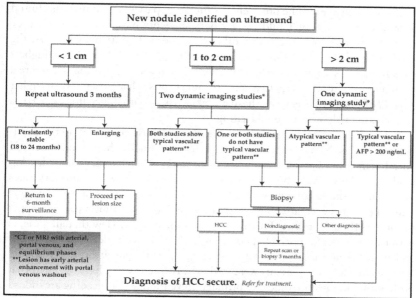

Figure 2-3. Guidelines for making diagnosis of HCC. (Based on the American Association for the Study of Liver Diseases recommendations found in Calle EE, Rodriguez C, Walker-Thurmond K, Thun MJ. Overweight, obesity, and mortality from cancer in a prospectively studied cohort of US adults. *N Engl J Med.* 2003;348:1625-1638.)

6 months with US and AFP) or enhanced (every 3 months, possibly using advanced imaging) follow-up, depending on the degree of suspicion.

ESOPHAGEAL VARICES

The development of esophageal varices (EVs) or gastric varices (GVs) is an ominous portent in patients with cirrhosis. In a systematic review of 118 studies on the natural progression of cirrhosis, patients with no ascites and no varices had a 1% yearly mortality rate, whereas those who had developed ascites and bleeding EVs had a 57% yearly mortality rate.[27] Initial studies indicated that each episode of bleeding from varices was associated with a 30% to 50% chance of death, but more recent studies have shown lower mortality rates in the 15% to 20% range per episode.[28] Despite the improvement noted in the care of EVs, the morbidity and mortality are high, and efforts to prevent bleeding EVs are clearly worthwhile.

EVs occur in the setting of portal hypertension, the most common cause of which is cirrhosis. In cirrhotic patients, EVs develop at a rate of approximately 8% per year,[29] and those with small varices will progress to large varices also at a rate of 8% per year. The prevalence is higher in patients with more profound liver disease—40% of Child's A cirrhotic patients have EVs, whereas they are found in 85% of those with Child's C cirrhosis. In patients with EVs, the yearly rate of bleeding from them ranges from 5% to 15%, with the highest rates in patients with large EVs.[30] Because EVs and bleeding from them are a consequence of portal hypertension, it is no surprise that patients with higher degrees of portal hypertension have a higher risk of initial bleeding, as well as an increased risk of recurrent bleeding.[31]

Etiologies of portal hypertension other than cirrhosis may result in the development of EVs. Noncirrhotic portal hypertension, Budd-Chiari syndrome, and portal vein thrombosis are examples of conditions wherein EVs may develop (and potentially bleed) but are not associated with the same mortality rates as seen in cirrhotic patients with EV bleeding. It is unclear whether the same screening and preventative measures used for EVs in cirrhotic patients apply to those without cirrhosis. This author takes the point of view that all patients with the potential for portal hypertension are at risk for the development of EVs and bleeding and that preventative strategies for the noncirrhotic EV should be employed as if the patients were cirrhotic. A recent study has suggested that both of the accepted methods for primary prevention of EV bleeding are indeed valid in a group of patients with EVs but no cirrhosis.[32]

Diagnosis of Esophageal Varices

The gold standard for the diagnosis of EVs or GVs is esophago-gastroduodenoscopy (EGD). Several size classifications have been used to describe EVs, but current recommendations are that the size classification be as simple as possible (ie, small or large). Small varices are considered low risk for bleeding, and thus preventative measures are not recommended, whereas large varices are at risk for rupture and primary prevention is indicated. Prophylactic trials using classification of EVs as "small," "medium," and "large" found that medium and large-sized EVs were at risk for bleeding.[30] When unclear from an EGD report, it is reasonable to err on the side of caution, either by obtaining a confirmatory study or simply electing to institute primary prophylaxis.

Because the point prevalence of significant (medium or large) EVs in cirrhotics is only 15% to 25%[33] efforts have been made to noninvasively predict the presence of EVs. Unfortunately, the predictive power for diagnosis of EVs with these noninvasive methods (including platelet count, spleen or portal vein size, and transient elastography) is insufficiently sensitive. As imaging technology improves, there has been increasing interest in modalities like CT for the diagnosis of EVs. A recent study found that CT was 90% sensitive and 50% specific in the detection of large varices.[34] In addition, CT had the added benefit of evaluating extraluminal pathology, and patients preferred it to EGD. It is unclear where CT (or other imaging) will ultimately fit into screening algorithms.

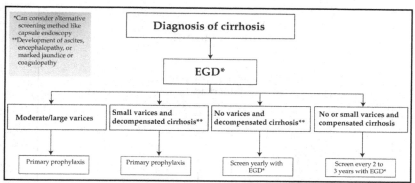

Figure 2-4. Varices screening and surveillance algorithm. (Based on the American Association for the Study of Liver Diseases guidelines found in Sarin SK, Gupta N, Jha SK, et al. Equal efficacy of endoscopic variceal ligation and propranolol in preventing variceal bleeding in patients with noncirrhotic portal hypertension. *Gastroenterology.* 2010;139:1238-1245.)

Lastly, a great deal of excitement has been generated for the use of capsule endoscopy for the detection of EVs. This procedure can be done without sedation and has recently been shown to have good operating characteristics, with a positive predictive value of 87% for differentiating large varices requiring treatment from small varices requiring continued surveillance.[35] EGD was clearly better at diagnosing EVs, making the diagnosis 15.6% more of the time, but the authors conclude that capsule endoscopy may be a good alternative to EGD given its minimal invasiveness and increased patient tolerance.

The natural history of EVs dictates the frequency with which patients with cirrhosis should have surveillance. **Current recommendations are that all patients with cirrhosis should receive an EGD to screen for varices once the diagnosis of cirrhosis is made.[33] If the diagnosis of medium or large EVs is made, then primary prophylaxis of EV bleeding should be initiated (below), and further surveillance for EVs is not necessary. Given that decompensated cirrhotics have the highest risk for developing varices, these patients should have surveillance EGDs yearly if they are found to have no or small varices on initial screen.** Patients with compensated cirrhosis and small varices on initial screen should undergo surveillance EGD every 1 to 2 years, and those with no varices on initial screen should undergo surveillance EGD every 2 to 3 years (Figure 2-4).

If significant varices are identified, treatment is warranted (Figure 2-5). For more detailed information on the treatment of varices, readers are referred to Chapter 4, "Management of Varices."

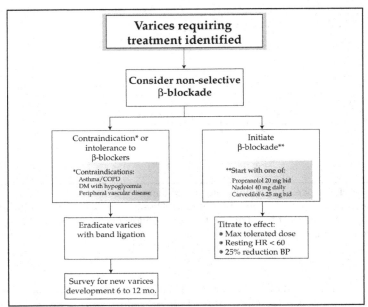

Figure 2-5. Primary prevention of bleeding in patients with varices. (Based on the American Association for the Study of Liver Diseases guidelines found in Sarin SK, Gupta N, Jha SK, et al. Equal efficacy of endoscopic variceal ligation and propranolol in preventing variceal bleeding in patients with noncirrhotic portal hypertension. *Gastroenterology.* 2010;139:1238-1245.)

BONE DISORDERS IN PATIENTS WITH CIRRHOSIS AND OTHER CHRONIC LIVER DISEASES

Bone disorders in patients with chronic liver disease have long been appreciated, especially in special populations including patients with cholestatic liver disease, post-liver transplantation patients, and patients on corticosteroids for the treatment of autoimmune hepatitis. More recent studies indicate that other forms of chronic liver disease are associated with osteoporosis and osteopenia.[36] The term *hepatic osteodystrophy* has been used to describe metabolic bone disorders in the context of chronic liver disease, but it is probably less confusing to simply use the more general terms of *osteoporosis, osteopenia*, and *osteomalacia*.

Osteoporosis is an absolute decrease in the amount of bone, whereas osteomalacia is a decrease in bone mineralization. Both disorders can lead to bone fragility and fractures. **Practically speaking, the primary bone disorder that occurs in patients with cirrhosis or other chronic liver disease is osteoporosis (and its more benign sibling osteopenia).** This is important to understand because the primary method for the diagnosis of bone disorders is bone densitometry with dual-energy X-ray absorptiometry (DXA), which shows reduced bone mineralization in both disorders. The gold standard for differentiating osteoporosis from osteomalacia is a bone biopsy, but the diagnosis of osteomalacia may be made with noninvasive testing in the setting of known risk factors (such as calcium malabsorption, syndromes of calcium or phosphate wasting, or insufficient vitamin D).[37] In the absence of such risk factors, patients with cirrhosis or other chronic liver disease and low bone density on DXA can reliably be given the diagnosis of osteoporosis.

In patients with cirrhosis listed for liver transplant, the prevalence of osteopenia and osteoporosis was 34.6% and 11.5%, respectively.[36] Patients with primary biliary cirrhosis (PBC) have an overall incidence of osteoporosis of 20% to 30% with a fracture rate of 7% to 14%, and those who have developed frank cirrhosis have an incidence over 40% and a fracture rate of 21%.[38] Patients with autoimmune hepatitis have significant bone loss, but it has been difficult to determine whether this is due to the liver disease or chronic immune suppression with corticosteroids.[39] Though there is an increased risk of osteoporosis in chronic liver disease as outlined above, the main risk for complications (atraumatic fractures) is immediately posttransplant. The primary risk factor for posttransplant fractures, however, is pretransplant osteopenia or osteoporosis.[40] Thus, it behooves all practitioners caring for patients with chronic liver disease to screen these populations and take preventative measures if significant bone loss is identified.

SCREENING FOR BONE DISEASE IN PATIENTS WITH CHRONIC LIVER DISEASE

Current recommendations suggest screening patients with chronic liver disease for bone disorders if they also have cholestatic liver disease, cirrhosis, or more than 3 months of corticosteroid treatment.[41] **To this list can be added patients with known fragility fractures (though an argument can be made for simply treating these patients, a baseline DXA can be useful to monitor treatment progress), postmenopausal women, and patients undergoing liver transplantation evaluation (who have not already been screened).**

For patients in the at-risk groups noted above who are found to have significant bone loss (osteoporosis), measures to prevent further bone loss and even build bone are indicated (Figure 2-6; see the Treatment section on p. 16). **For at-risk patients who have normal bone density on screening DXA, they should be entered into a surveillance program of DXA scans every 2 to 3 years, with the exception of those patients on chronic corticosteroids, who should get a DXA screening every year.**

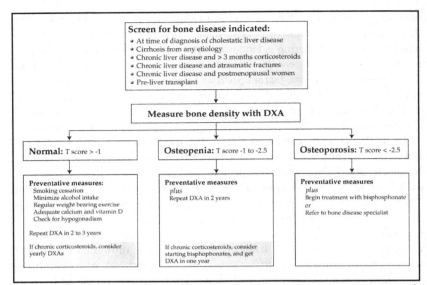

Figure 2-6. Screening and treatment algorithm for osteoporosis in patients with chronic liver disease. (Based on American Gastroenterological Association guidelines found in Carey EJ, Balan V, Kremers WK, Hay JE. Osteopenia and osteoporosis in patients with end-stage liver disease caused by hepatitis C and alcoholic liver disease: not just a cholestatic problem. *Liver Transpl.* 2003;9:1166-1173.)

TREATMENT OF OSTEOPOROSIS IN PATIENTS WITH CHRONIC LIVER DISEASE

Patients with cirrhosis or cholestatic liver diseases should be checked for vitamin D deficiency, with repletion for those deficient. Calcium supplementation should be the standard of care for patients with cholestatic liver disease because malabsorption of calcium is common in these patients. In addition, general measures to promote good bone health should be discussed with the patient, including smoking cessation, minimization of alcohol use, and regular weight-bearing exercises.

Hormonal therapy for prevention and treatment of bone loss is controversial, and benefits must be weighed against known risks. Females with chronic liver disease may undergo early menopause (< 45 years old), and if they develop osteoporosis, estrogens may be indicated, again weighing the known risks of this therapy. Selective estrogen receptor modulators may be used in this context as well. For males with hypogonadism and low testosterone levels, treatment with testosterone for prevention of osteoporosis development is reasonable.

Bisphosphonates are generally safe in patients with chronic liver disease and may be considered first-line therapy in patients with

osteoporosis or osteopenia. Other therapies such as calcitonin and parathyroid hormone may be considered in this population but probably should be prescribed with the input of a bone disease specialist. Fluoride is not recommended for the treatment or prevention of bone disease in patients with hepatic disease. Given the difficulties of managing osteoporosis in the context of chronic liver disease, it is often helpful to involve a bone disease specialist when screening identifies significant bone disease in these already complex patients.

REFERENCES

1. Sangiovanni A, Del Ninno E, Fasani P, et al. Increased survival of cirrhotic patients with a hepatocellular carcinoma detected during surveillance. *Gastroenterology.* 2004;126:1005-1014.
2. Benvegnu L, Gios M, Boccato S, Alberti A. Natural history of compensated viral cirrhosis: a prospective study on the incidence and hierarchy of major complications. *Gut.* 2004;53:744-749.
3. Llovet JM, Burroughs A, Bruix J. Hepatocellular carcinoma. *Lancet.* 2003;362:1907-1917.
4. El-Serag HB, Mason AC. Rising incidence of hepatocellular carcinoma in the United States. *N Engl J Med.* 1999;340:745-750.
5. Parkin DM, Bray F, Ferlay J, Pisani P. Estimating the world cancer burden: Globocan 2000. *Int J Cancer.* 2001;94:153-156.
6. Bosch FX, Ribes J, Diaz M, Cleries R. Primary liver cancer: worldwide incidence and trends. *Gastroenterology.* 2004;127(5 suppl 1):S5-S16.
7. Fattovich G, Stroffolini T, Zagni I, Donato F. Hepatocellular carcinoma in cirrhosis: incidence and risk factors. *Gastroenterology.* 2004;127(5 suppl 1):S35-S50.
8. Lavanchy D. Hepatitis B virus epidemiology, disease burden, treatment, and current and emerging prevention and control measures. *J Viral Hepat.* 2004;11:97-107.
9. Chang MH, Chen CJ, Lai MS, et al. Universal hepatitis B vaccination in Taiwan and the incidence of hepatocellular carcinoma in children. Taiwan Childhood Hepatoma Study Group. *N Engl J Med.* 1997;336:1855-1859.
10. Lee MS, Kim DH, Kim H, et al. Hepatitis B vaccination and reduced risk of primary liver cancer among male adults: a cohort study in Korea. *Int J Epidemiol.* 1998;27:316-319.
11. Stroffolini T, Mele A, Tosti ME, et al. The impact of the hepatitis B mass immunisation campaign on the incidence and risk factors of acute hepatitis B in Italy. *J Hepatol.* 2000;33:980-985.
12. Freeman AJ, Dore GJ, Law MG, et al. Estimating progression to cirrhosis in chronic hepatitis C virus infection. *Hepatology.* 2001;34(4 Pt 1):809-816.
13. El-Serag HB, Rudolph KL. Hepatocellular carcinoma: epidemiology and molecular carcinogenesis. *Gastroenterology.* 2007;132:2557-2576.
14. Kowdley KV. Iron, hemochromatosis, and hepatocellular carcinoma. *Gastroenterology.* 2004;127(5 suppl 1):S79-S86.
15. El-Serag HB, Tran T, Everhart JE. Diabetes increases the risk of chronic liver disease and hepatocellular carcinoma. *Gastroenterology.* 2004;126:460-468.
16. Caldwell SH, Crespo DM, Kang HS, Al-Osaimi AM. Obesity and hepatocellular carcinoma. *Gastroenterology.* 2004;127(5 suppl 1):S97-S103.
17. Morgan TR, Mandayam S, Jamal MM. Alcohol and hepatocellular carcinoma. *Gastroenterology.* 2004;127(5 suppl 1):S87-S96.
18. Hashimoto E, Yatsuji S, Tobari M, et al. Hepatocellular carcinoma in patients with nonalcoholic steatohepatitis. *J Gastroenterol.* 2009;44(suppl 19):89-95.
19. Calle EE, Rodriguez C, Walker-Thurmond K, Thun MJ. Overweight, obesity, and mortality from cancer in a prospectively studied cohort of US adults. *N Engl J Med.* 2003;348:1625-1638.
20. Bruix J, Sherman M. Management of hepatocellular carcinoma. *Hepatology.* 2005;42:1208-1236.
21. Mazzaferro V, Regalia E, Doci R, et al. Liver transplantation for the treatment of small hepatocellular carcinomas in patients with cirrhosis. *N Engl J Med.* 1996;334:693-699.
22. Nathan H, Schulick RD, Choti MA, Pawlik TM. Predictors of survival after resection of early hepatocellular carcinoma. *Ann Surg.* 2009;249:799-805.

23. Mazzaferro V, Llovet JM, Miceli R, et al. Predicting survival after liver transplantation in patients with hepatocellular carcinoma beyond the Milan criteria: a retrospective, exploratory analysis. *Lancet Oncol.* 2009;10:35-43.

24. Hiraoka A, Horiike N, Yamashita Y, et al. Efficacy of radiofrequency ablation therapy compared to surgical resection in 164 patients in Japan with single hepatocellular carcinoma smaller than 3 cm, along with report of complications. *Hepatogastroenterology.* 2008;55:2171-2174.

25. Gupta S, Bent S, Kohlwes J. Test characteristics of alpha-fetoprotein for detecting hepatocellular carcinoma in patients with hepatitis C. A systematic review and critical analysis. *Ann Intern Med.* 2003;139:46-50.

26. Colli A, Fraquelli M, Casazza G, et al. Accuracy of ultrasonography, spiral CT, magnetic resonance, and alpha-fetoprotein in diagnosing hepatocellular carcinoma: a systematic review. *Am J Gastroenterol.* 2006;101:513-523.

27. D'Amico G, Garcia-Tsao G, Pagliaro L. Natural history and prognostic indicators of survival in cirrhosis: a systematic review of 118 studies. *J Hepatol.* 2006;44:217-231.

28. Chalasani N, Kahi C, Francois F, et al. Improved patient survival after acute variceal bleeding: a multicenter, cohort study. *Am J Gastroenterol.* 2003;98:653-659.

29. Zhao C, Chen SB, Zhou JP, et al. Prognosis of hepatic cirrhosis patients with esophageal or gastric variceal hemorrhage: multivariate analysis. *Hepatobiliary Pancreat Dis Int.* 2002;1:416-419.

30. North Italian Endoscopic Club for the Study and Treatment of Esophageal Varices. Prediction of the first variceal hemorrhage in patients with cirrhosis of the liver and esophageal varices. A prospective multicenter study. *N Engl J Med.* 1988;319:983-989.

31. Feu F, García-Pagán JC, Bosch J, et al. Relation between portal pressure response to pharmacotherapy and risk of recurrent variceal haemorrhage in patients with cirrhosis. *Lancet.* 1995;346:1056-1059.

32. Sarin SK, Gupta N, Jha SK, et al. Equal efficacy of endoscopic variceal ligation and propranolol in preventing variceal bleeding in patients with noncirrhotic portal hypertension. *Gastroenterology.* 2010;139:1238-1245.

33. Garcia-Tsao G, Sanyal AJ, Grace ND, Carey W; Practice Guidelines Committee of the American Association for the Study of Liver Diseases; Practice Parameters Committee of the American College of Gastroenterology. Prevention and management of gastroesophageal varices and variceal hemorrhage in cirrhosis. *Hepatology.* 2007;46:922-938.

34. Perri RE, Chiorean MV, Fidler JL, et al. A prospective evaluation of computerized tomographic (CT) scanning as a screening modality for esophageal varices. *Hepatology.* 2008;47:1587-1594.

35. de Franchis R, Eisen GM, Laine L, et al. Esophageal capsule endoscopy for screening and surveillance of esophageal varices in patients with portal hypertension. *Hepatology.* 2008;47:1595-1603.

36. Sokhi RP, Anantharaju A, Kondaveeti R, et al. Bone mineral density among cirrhotic patients awaiting liver transplantation. *Liver Transpl.* 2004;10:648-653.

37. Bingham CT, Fitzpatrick LA. Noninvasive testing in the diagnosis of osteomalacia. *Am J Med.* 1993;95:519-523.

38. Hay JE, Guichelaar MM. Evaluation and management of osteoporosis in liver disease. *Clin Liver Dis.* 2005;9:747-766, viii.

39. Stellon AJ, Davies A, Compston J, Williams R. Bone loss in autoimmune chronic active hepatitis on maintenance corticosteroid therapy. *Gastroenterology.* 1985;89:1078-1083.

40. Carey EJ, Balan V, Kremers WK, Hay JE. Osteopenia and osteoporosis in patients with end-stage liver disease caused by hepatitis C and alcoholic liver disease: not just a cholestatic problem. *Liver Transpl.* 2003;9:1166-1173.

41. Leslie WD, Bernstein CN, Leboff MS; the American Gastroenterological Association Clinical Practice Committee. AGA technical review on osteoporosis in hepatic disorders. *Gastroenterology.* 2003;125:941-966.

NUTRITION IN PATIENTS WITH CIRRHOSIS

Anna Sasaki, MD, PhD

One of the most pervasive and neglected issues confronting the clinician caring for a cirrhotic patient is that of malnutrition. Estimates of clinically significant inpatient malnutrition vary from 60% to 90% and occur irrespective of the etiology of the liver disease.[1-3] The consequences of malnutrition in patients with chronic liver disease affect not only the patients but also result in higher in-hospital mortality, greater length of stay, and higher costs.[4] In addition, there is a correlation between the severity of the liver disease and the degree of malnutrition.

In the 19th and early 20th centuries, cirrhosis in the alcoholic was termed *nutritional cirrhosis* and the approach was to provide the patients with high-quality protein calories as well as promote the maintenance of abstinence. An Internet search revealed that even today for the lay public, portal cirrhosis is defined as nutritional cirrhosis and is distinguished from congestive, biliary, and postnecrotic cirrhosis. After the Rubin and Lieber study showing that baboons could develop hepatic fibrosis if they ingested alcohol with an adequate diet,[5] the focus on etiology shifted to alcohol as the primary etiology of cirrhosis. Also, nutritional deficiencies per se probably do not cause cirrhosis in humans, but they do contribute to hepatic dysfunction.[6] Conversely, cirrhosis accelerates the development of malnutrition, as will be seen.

The original classification of surgical risk due to cirrhosis by C. G. Child in 1964 included nutrition as a variable. The subsequent modifications removed

Zaman A. *Managing the Complications of Cirrhosis: A Practical Approach* (pp 19-28).

nutrition because of its subjective nature, and the model for end-stage liver disease (MELD) score, used to predict outcomes in patients with liver disease, also does not take nutrition into account. As a result, patients are frequently referred for liver transplant evaluation because they are significantly muscle-wasted and weak. Unfortunately, they do not have a MELD score high enough to qualify for transplant because the liver dysfunction itself is not severe. This can result in frustration for the patient, the family, and sometimes the referring providers, who feel that their loved ones or patients are dying but not being offered a life-saving therapy. There is a high mortality on the waiting list of this subset of patients, and frequently there is a recent history of hospitalization or prolonged inability to take in food. The challenge in cirrhotic patients in general is to minimize iatrogenic reasons for malnutrition. In the subset of patients afflicted with malnutrition and muscle wasting, it is difficult and sometimes futile to try to reverse the process. The patients have poor appetite, fatigue when eating, and minimal ability to exercise. Thus, the goal should always be the prevention of malnutrition.

One of the fastest growing causes of cirrhosis and decompensated liver disease is related to nonalcoholic steatohepatitis. These patients are often obese and suffer from Type 2 diabetes and/or hyperlipidemia. Patients with nonalcoholic steatohepatitis or alcoholic liver disease have a 25% prevalence of malnutrition (by body mass index [BMI]) on admission to the hospital, whereas 75% of those with other forms of liver disease are malnourished.[3] This underscores the concept that patients may be malnourished while still maintaining body mass. These patients, however, may also be protein malnourished and vitamin deficient.[7] This seemingly paradoxical finding may be because their body fat was maintained even while muscle atrophy was occurring. Many transplant centers defer patients from transplant listing until their BMI is less than 35 because of the comorbidities associated with diabetes and obesity.[8] The challenge in these patients is to achieve effective weight loss while maintaining adequate protein intake. The team approach is particularly important in these patients, involving the patient, the family, the medical provider, dietitians, and social workers. At times, mental health providers and endocrinology specialists also need to provide input.

SPECIFIC NUTRITIONAL ISSUES

There are many factors that contribute to malnutrition in the cirrhotic patient (Table 3-1). Food may be unpalatable due to dietary restriction of salt (to decrease fluid retention) and sugar (in diabetics), and the patient may have early satiety due to tense ascites. The cirrhotic patient may experience fatigue, either of muscles used for chewing or a decreased ability to remain upright for a sufficient amount of time to take in an adequate amount of food. The taste of the food is changed also, due partly to neurotoxins and partly to abnormal

---
Table 3-1

Causes of Malnutrition in Cirrhosis

Diets restricted in salt, sugar, protein	Unpalatable
Hospitalization	Nothing by mouth for tests, procedures
	Anorexia because of underlying illness
Ascites	Early satiety
Abnormal macronutrient metabolism	↑ protein oxidation, ↓ synthesis
	Glucose
	Fat
Deficiencies in vitamins, minerals	Alteration in taste; anemias
Encephalopathy	Forgets to eat; alteration in taste
Socioeconomic issues	Decreased access to nutritious foods
Pulmonary excretion of sulfur metabolites	Alteration in taste
Muscle weakness	Fatigue with chewing
Cultural issues	Meals 1 to 2 times a day

---

excretion of sulfur metabolites. Anorexia may occur due to recurrent infections, other underlying illnesses, or depression. A patient affected by even minimal encephalopathy may forget to eat or may not be capable of fixing a meal. These factors may exist to varying degrees in cirrhotic patients, but all cirrhotics have changes in protein and energy metabolism.[9]

The resting energy expenditure in cirrhotic patients may be high, low, or normal depending on the stability of their medical condition, the presence of infection or inflammation, and the degree of malnutrition. In advanced liver disease, the respiratory quotient is in the 0.6 to 0.7 range and resembles that of hypermetabolism. Negative nitrogen balance, lower body cell mass, and decreased fat and glycogen stores are common.[10,11] Serum levels of catecholamines and endotoxins are higher.

Because of portal hypertension and shunting of nutrient-rich blood from the gut to the systemic circulation, there is a decrease in the first-pass uptake of glucose and amino acids by the liver. There may also be a decrease in lipoprotein synthesis, affecting lipid transport and metabolism. Peripheral serum levels of nutrients are higher and there is a mismatch between hepatic uptake and pancreatic hormone secretions. There is a shift in metabolism in the cirrhotic from carbohydrate to fat metabolism after an overnight fast (12 to 14 hours) such that cirrhotics derive 75% of their energy from fat, whereas healthy people derive only 35% of their calorie needs from fat.[10] Normal controls take an average of 2 to 3 days to shift their metabolism to fat utilization.

Protein handling and utilization are significantly altered in patients with cirrhosis, even in those with normal liver function parameters. There is increased protein oxidation as amino acids are broken down for fuel by the liver. There is accelerated protein breakdown as systemic protein needs are altered, but there is inefficient protein resynthesis.

Glucose metabolism is also altered because insulin is not appropriately degraded by the liver. These patients develop hyperinsulinemia, insulin resistance, and consequent glucose intolerance, leading to the shift to fat as fuel.

Lipid metabolism, however, is also affected because of both the release of triglyceride by the adipocytes and the decrease in apolipoprotein synthesis and lipoprotein conjugation in the hepatocytes. Arachidonic acid may be deficient, and the cholesterol–phospholipid ratio in cell membranes may be increased, resulting in changes in membrane fluidity.

Micronutrient deficiencies are common in patients with cirrhosis. Whereas many water-soluble vitamin deficiencies (folate, pyridoxine, vitamin C) are associated with alcoholic liver disease, patients with nonalcoholic cirrhosis may also be deficient in water-soluble as well as fat-soluble vitamins. The disruption of enterohepatic circulation can lead to abnormal utilization of folate and B_{12}. Thiamine has been shown to be decreased in patients with hepatitis C cirrhosis.[12] The serum levels of lipid-soluble vitamins are frequently decreased in patients with cholestatic liver diseases such as primary biliary cirrhosis and primary sclerosing cholangitis; these levels should be routinely assessed in these patients. In addition, up to 40% of patients with noncholestatic liver diseases may have deficiencies in vitamin A.[13] Vitamin K may be deficient in cirrhotics given repeated courses of antibiotics. Vitamin D levels are often low in patients with cirrhosis, and the levels are correlated with the severity of the liver disease. Osteoporosis is common in patients referred for liver transplant, irrespective of the etiology of the liver disease. Possible causes include lack of outdoor activity, decreased intake, relative malabsorption, as well as decreased hydroxylation by the liver.

Assessment of nutritional status in the patient with decompensated cirrhosis is fraught with difficulties. Serum levels of albumin, pre-albumin, and transferrin, all synthesized by the liver, may be diminished. The serum creatinine may be low or high, depending on the degree of renal dysfunction, and will affect the creatinine-height index. Muscle wasting may be masked by obesity. The subjective global assessment has been validated in patients with decompensated cirrhosis[14,15] and is probably the easiest to administer at the bedside. The premise is that the history and physical provide an accurate assessment of the degree of malnutrition, taking into account weight change, changes in dietary intake, the presence or absence of gastrointestinal symptoms, and the physical findings of muscle atrophy and loss of subcutaneous fat.[16] Other, multicompartmental analyses may be more sensitive but are cumbersome.

```
┌──────────────────────────────────────────────────────────────────────┐
│                          ALGORITHM I                                    │
│         Subjective Global Assessment of Nutrition—INPATIENT             │
│                                                                          │
│        Mild                  Moderate                  Severe            │
│   Calorie counts          Calorie counts           Tube feeding         │
│   Nutrition education     Tube feeding within      within 48 hours      │
│   Consider tube feeding   2 to 3 days              Correct underlying causes │
│   4 to 5 days                                      TPN only as last resort  │
│                                                    (see text)            │
└──────────────────────────────────────────────────────────────────────┘
```

TREATMENT ALGORITHM I— INPATIENT NUTRITION SUPPORT

Because most cirrhotic patients requiring inpatient care are moderately to severely malnourished, a high level of awareness on the part of the provider is needed to ensure nutritional repletion. Such patients should go no longer than 24 to 48 hours without adequate nutrition. The most common cause of failure to provide a patient with adequate nutrition is the need to keep patients from ingesting anything by mouth (NPO) for tests and procedures. A second cause is concern that enteral or oral feeding may disrupt therapeutic bands after variceal bleeding with band ligation. Although there is controversy in the literature, the approach taken by the Royal Free Hospital is felt to be safe: the patient is kept NPO for 24 hours after band ligation, and then oral or enteral nutrition is resumed. When the local standard of care is to feed the patients only liquids for 24 to 48 hours following banding of varices, adequate liquid nutrition in the form of standardized formulas with protein supplementation as needed is appropriate and well tolerated.

The diet prescription advocated in the literature[1,17] is a low-salt diet (< 2000 mg/day), with high protein (1.2 to 1.5 g/kg/day), and with frequent small feedings—as many as 6 per day. It has been shown that patients are more likely to achieve a positive nitrogen balance when given a protein-rich bedtime snack.[9] In the most severely malnourished patients, up to 1.8 g/kg/day protein intake is associated with increased probability of positive nitrogen balance (Algorithm I).[17]

Inpatients seldom ingest the amount of calories and protein that they need, but even more seldom do they begin enteral nutrition in a timely fashion. It has been shown that patients tolerate tube placement and feeding much better if the providers discuss the importance of enteral nutrition in a positive and enthusiastic manner. Nausea is not a contraindication to enteral feeding, particularly if the tube can be passed beyond the pylorus. **One of the barriers** to adequate enteral feeding is the stoppage of the tube feed when the patient is taken to radiology, physical therapy, or other hospital locations. Vigilance is needed to ensure that the patient receives as close to 100% of the prescribed dose of nutrition as possible.

Total parenteral nutrition (TPN) should be prescribed only as a last resort in patients who have absolute contraindications to enteral feeding. Examples of this are prolonged ileus, intestinal ischemia, severe malabsorption, and high likelihood of aspiration of tube feeding material. TPN will not replete the patient's malnourished state faster or more completely than enteral nutrition, and the risk of infection, particularly high in decompensated cirrhotics, leads to increased morbidity and mortality. Standard amino acid, glucose, and lipid solutions are effective in improving nutritional parameters if TPN is indicated.

TREATMENT ALGORITHM II— OUTPATIENT NUTRITION SUPPORT

It is much more difficult in the outpatient setting to obtain adherence to the liver-healthy diet. Many adults, particularly in the United States, eat only dinner, although they may snack afterwards. A cirrhotic patient with this approach may spend a significant amount of time with the metabolic shift that promotes muscle catabolism. In addition, outpatients in particular need to be educated about the need for a high protein diet. Many have been told by their primary providers or have read on the Internet that ingested protein causes encephalopathy. Others have heard that vegetable protein is acceptable but one should avoid animal protein. Finally, some patients and their caregivers try to eat a heart-healthy diet—a low-fat, high-complex-carbohydrate diet with many servings of fruits and vegetables. **There is almost uniform agreement that ingested protein does not precipitate encephalopathy in the patient with decompensated cirrhosis; in fact, as described above, cirrhotic patients need at least 1.5 times the amount of protein per pound of body weight per day that a normal person needs.** The type of protein is less important; however, meat protein is more bio-available and is up to 95% absorbed by the small bowel, whereas vegetable protein is absorbed only 45% to 60% due to binding to fiber and consequent lack of availability to digestive enzymes. As long as the patient is having frequent soft stools, meat protein is safe and often considered by the patient to be more consistent with his or her premorbid normal diet (Algorithm II).

As important as what is eaten is the frequency of food intake. Whereas the normal person develops the metabolic shift of starvation after 2 to 3 days of lack of food intake, the cirrhotic patient begins to develop this shift after

---

ALGORITHM II

Subjective Global Assessment of Nutrition—OUTPATIENT

Mild	*Moderate*	*Severe*
Nutritional education:	Food diaries	Tube feeding
High protein	Dietary consult	Search for other causes
(1.2 to 1.5 g/kg/d)	Social service consult	
Frequent small meals		
Low salt		

---

12 to 14 hours. **Frequent small feedings, such as recommended in the diabetic diet, can provide adequate calories and protein, is better tolerated by patients with ascites or muscle wasting, and will prevent the metabolic shifts that result in further muscle wasting.**
Dietitians should be consulted early in the course of the cirrhotic patient's decline to help the patient and caregivers maintain adequate nutrient intake. A food diary over the course of a week can provide information to the dietitian as to the type and frequency of food intake. Liquid supplements may be better tolerated than solid protein and, in general, homemade shakes and smoothies are more nutritious and less expensive than commercially prepared ones. The advantage of the latter, of course, is the ease of preparation, particularly when the patient has to prepare the meals.

WHAT IF THE TREATMENT ALGORITHM IS INEFFECTIVE?

If the treatment algorithms are ineffective in the inpatient setting, one must first ensure that the patient is actually receiving all of the nutrition prescribed. If so, causes of hypermetabolism, such as covert infection or intermittent endotoxemia, or causes of increased protein loss, such as malabsorption or protein-losing nephropathy or enteropathy, must be sought. It is possible, though, in a severely malnourished Child's C cirrhotic, that there is a point of irreversibility, such that no nutrition will improve the patient's nutritional parameters. The prognosis in this situation is very poor, and the patient may be deemed too sick to survive transplantation.

In the outpatient setting, similar investigation may be revealing. It is essential to ensure that there are no barriers to buying, preparing, or eating the food. Social workers may need to be consulted to explore ways to ensure that patients have access to food. If it becomes clear, usually through a decline in liver function labs, that the liver dysfunction itself is the source of the malnutrition, expedited transplant referral is appropriate.

Table 3-2

Possible Positive Outcomes of Improvement in Nutrition in Patients With Cirrhosis

- Promote hepatic regeneration
- Prevent or decrease protein breakdown
- Prevent shift to fat metabolism
- Decrease production of stress hormones
- Improve immune function
- Improve tissue growth and repair
- Avoid macro- and micronutrient deficiencies
- Decrease morbidity and mortality
- Improve the patient's sense of well-being

Referral for transplant evaluation in the appropriate patient should occur before there is clinical evidence of malnutrition. Unfortunately, patients may have medical or psychosocial barriers to transplantation that need to be addressed before they can be accepted, and their condition may deteriorate during that time. In addition, patients may present for medical attention only when malnutrition is far advanced. Finally, patients may have absolute contraindications to transplant. The degree of malnutrition allows the provider to counsel the patient and family regarding the prognosis.

In summary, the provider should assume that all patients with cirrhosis are malnourished to some degree due to changes in nutrient ingestion, absorption, and utilization. Early multidisciplinary intervention and aggressive repletion of nutrient deficiencies can prevent the downward spiral that afflicts many patients with decompensated cirrhosis. Possible positive outcomes of this approach are listed in Table 3-2, the most important of which are the improvement in morbidity and mortality and in the patient's sense of well-being.

REFERENCES

1. O'Brien A, Williams R. Nutrition in end-stage liver disease: principles and practice. *Gastroenterology.* 2008;134:1729-1740.
2. Campillo B, Richardet JP, Scherman E, Bories PN. Evaluation of nutritional practice in hospitalized cirrhotic patients: results of a prospective study. *Nutrition.* 2003;19:515-521.
3. Sarin SK, Dhingra N, Bansal A, Malhotra S, Guptan RC. Dietary and nutritional abnormalities in alcoholic liver disease: a comparison with chronic alcoholics without liver disease. *Am J Gastroenterol.* 1997;92:777-783.
4. Sam J, Nguyen GC. Protein–calorie malnutrition as a prognostic indicator of mortality among patients hospitalized with cirrhosis and portal hypertension. *Liver Int.* 2009;29:1396-1402.
5. Rubin E, Lieber CS. Experimental alcoholic hepatitis: a new primate model. *Science.* 1973;182:712-713.

6. Popper H, Schaffner F. Nutritional cirrhosis in man? *N Engl J Med.* 1971;285:577-578.

7. Aasheim ET, Hofsø D, Hjelmesaeth J, Birkeland KI, Bøhmer T. Vitamin status in morbidly obese patients: a cross-sectional study. *Am J Clin Nutr.* 2008;87:362-369.

8. Hasse J. Pretransplant obesity: a weighty issue affecting transplant candidacy and outcomes. *Nutr Clin Pract.* 2007;22:494-504.

9. Richardson R, Sutherland D, Garden OJ. Macronutrient preference, dietary intake, and substrate oxidation among stable cirrhotic patients. *Hepatology.* 1999;29:1380-1386.

10. Kondrup J, Mueller MJ. Energy and protein requirements of patients with chronic liver disease. *J Hepatol.* 1997;27:239-247.

11. Davidson HI, Riggio O, Merli M, et al. Early postprandial energy expenditure and macronutrient use after a mixed meal in cirrhotic patients. *JPEN J Parenter Enteral Nutr.* 1992;16:445-450.

12. Lévy S, Hervé C, Delacoux E, Erlinger S. Thiamine deficiency in hepatitis C virus and alcohol-related liver diseases. *Dig Dis Sci.* 2002;47:543-548.

13. Ukleja A, Scolapio JS, McConnell JP, et al. Nutritional assessment of serum and hepatic vitamin A levels in patients with cirrhosis. *JPEN J Parenter Enteral Nutr.* 2002;26:184-188.

14. Hasse JM. Diet therapy for organ transplantation. A problem-based approach. *Nurs Clin North Am.* 1997;32:863-880.

15. Hasse J, Strong S, Gorman MA, Liepa G. Subjective global assessment: alternative nutrition-assessment technique for liver-transplant candidates. *Nutrition.* 1993;9:339-343.

16. Baker JP, Detsky AS, Whitwell J, Langer B, Jeejeebhoy KN. A comparison of the predictive value of nutritional assessment techniques. *Hum Nutr Clin Nutr.* 1982;36:233-241.

17. Wohl D, Falck-Ytter Y, McCullough AJ. Nutrition in Liver Disease. *Clinical Perspectives in Gastroenterology.* 1999;2:267-74.

chapter

MANAGEMENT OF VARICES

Edoardo G. Giannini, MD, PhD, FACG

PATHOPHYSIOLOGY, PREVALENCE, AND INCIDENCE OF ESOPHAGEAL VARICES

Development of esophageal varices (EVs) in patients with compensated cirrhosis marks a change from a clinical stage with a very low risk of death at 1 year (1% risk) to an intermediate-risk stage (3.4% risk at 1 year).[1] Furthermore, variceal hemorrhage indicates the transition from a compensated to a decompensated stage of disease with a very high 1-year risk of death (57% risk) and accounts for approximately one-third of all deaths among patients with chronic liver disease and cirrhosis.[1] Mortality from variceal bleeding decreased during the last decades due to advances achieved in its treatment, although a bleeding episode still carries a mortality rate of up to 20% within 6 weeks.[2]

Pathophysiology

Variceal formation and bleeding are strictly related to the presence and degree of portal hypertension. In cirrhotic patients, portal pressure increases mainly because of the combination of 2 pathophysiological events:

- Increased resistance to the passage of blood through the liver due to architectural distortion resulting from fibrosis, regenerative nodules, and intrahepatic vasoconstriction;
- Splanchnic arteriolar vascular bed vasodilatation leading to increased portal venous blood inflow.

Zaman A. *Managing the Complications of Cirrhosis: A Practical Approach* (pp 29-60).

Table 4-1

Prevalence and Incidence of Esophageal Varices

	Prevalence (%)
Compensated cirrhosis	30 to 50
Decompensated cirrhosis	> 80
	Incidence (% per year)
No varices → small varices	5 to 10
Small varices → large varices	5 to 30

Portal pressure is a product of portal inflow and outflow resistance (Portal pressure = Portal venous inflow × Resistance to portal venous outflow). A reliable indicator of portal pressure can be invasively determined by catheterization of the hepatic vein through a transfemoral or transjugular access and measurement of both free hepatic venous pressure (FHVP) and wedged hepatic venous pressure (WHVP). The hepatic venous pressure gradient (HVPG) provides an indirect but precise estimate of the portal pressure and can be calculated by subtracting the FHVP from the WHVP (HVPG = WHVP – FHVP). Normal HVPG is 3 to 5 mm Hg, and an elevation of the HVPG to greater than 5 mm Hg denotes portal hypertension.[3] When portal pressure increases and portal hypertension occurs, the obstacle to portal blood inflow is partially compensated for by an increase in blood flow through porto-collateral communications such as veins around the gastroesophageal junction, which eventually become dilated and form EVs. It has been shown that varices do not form and bleed at an HVPG below 10 to 12 mm Hg, and an increase of HVPG above a 10-mm Hg threshold is defined as clinically significant portal hypertension.[3,4] Because HVPG measurement is not widely available in many centers, from the practical standpoint, the presence of varices, variceal hemorrhage, and/or ascites is indicative of the presence of clinically significant portal hypertension.[5]

Prevalence and Incidence of Varices

Knowledge of the prevalence, rate of development, and progression in size from small to large of EVs is important because it may help plan surveillance endoscopy intervals and assess the bleeding risk of cirrhotic patients (Table 4-1). The prevalence of EVs increases with worsening of the underlying liver disease, ranging from 50% in Child-Pugh class A patients to more than 80% in Child-Pugh class C patients.[6] In patients without EVs at screening endoscopy, varices tend to develop at a yearly rate of 5% to 10%.[7] In patients without varices, the presence of an HVPG > 10 mm Hg at the time of initial screening endoscopy doubles the risk of developing EVs compared to patients with an HVPG below this threshold (50% versus 25% at 5-year follow-up) and is the strongest predictor of varices development.[8] If HVPG cannot be measured, thrombocytopenia and an increase in Child-Pugh score can be used as surrogate markers because they have been associated with an increased risk of developing varices.[9] In patients with small varices at initial endoscopy, post-alcoholic origin of liver disease, Child-Pugh class B or C, and the presence of red wale marks (longitudinal, dilated venules resembling whip marks on the variceal surface) have been identified as independent predictors of the growth in size of varices.[7] On the average, the yearly progression rate ranges between 15% and 30%.[10] Gastric varices are less prevalent than EVs and are present in 5% to 33% of cirrhotic patients with portal hypertension. Although gastric varices account for about 10% of all portal hypertension-related bleedings, the bleeding risk of gastric varices is about 25% at 2 years.[11] The main risk factors for gastric variceal bleeding are their location and size (fundal and larger varices are more likely to bleed) the presence of decompensated liver disease (Child-Pugh class B or C), and the endoscopic presence of red spots (localized reddish mucosal areas or spots on the surface of a varix). The prevalence of portal hypertensive gastropathy ranges from 9% to 57%, depending on patient selection and variability in the criteria used for diagnosis and classification.[12] The main factors associated with the presence of portal hypertensive gastropathy are portal hypertension and severity of liver disease,[13] although both the presence and severity of portal hypertensive gastropathy do not have a linear correlation with the severity of portal hypertension.[12] It is still debated whether endoscopic obliteration of EVs may be associated with development or worsening of portal hypertensive gastropathy. The frequency of acute bleeding from portal hypertensive gastropathy is difficult to estimate because chronic bleeding with gradual development of iron-deficient anemia is most likely to occur, and mortality associated with bleeding from portal hypertensive gastropathy is low.[12,13]

DIAGNOSIS AND CLASSIFICATION OF VARICES

Screening and Surveillance

The only adequate method for diagnosing and grading EVs is upper digestive endoscopy, because it also allows for identification and staging of gastric varices and portal hypertensive gastropathy. **All cirrhotic patients should undergo initial endoscopic screening for EVs at the time of diagnosis of cirrhosis because endoscopy helps stratify patients according to their risk of bleeding on the basis of variceal size and appearance and identifies patients who can benefit from prophylactic treatment aimed at reducing the likelihood of bleeding (Figure 4-1).[14,15]**

Patients without varices at screening endoscopy should be followed up with surveillance endoscopies to detect the appearance of large varices.

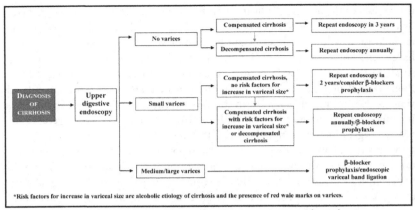

*Risk factors for increase in variceal size are alcoholic etiology of cirrhosis and the presence of red wale marks on varices.

Figure 4-1. Screening and surveillance for EVs in patients with cirrhosis.

Compensated patients without varices at screening endoscopy can repeat endoscopy at a 3-year interval and at clinical decompensation, whereas decompensated patients should repeat endoscopy annually (see Figure 4-1).[14,15]

Patients with small varices without risk factors for increase in variceal size (ie, alcoholic origin of cirrhosis, Child-Pugh class B or C, and red signs on varices) should be re-endoscoped at a 2-year interval, and patients with any of the above-mentioned risk factors in whom the increase in variceal size appears to be faster and there is an increased risk of bleeding should be re-endoscoped at 1-year intervals.[14,15] **Alternatively, prophylaxis can be started when risk factors for increase in size and bleeding are present (see Figure 4-1).**

Patients diagnosed with large varices should start prophylactic therapy to prevent variceal hemorrhage (see Figure 4-1).[14,15]

Endoscopic Classification of Varices

EVs are classified by size and presence of endoscopic features, because these 2 characteristics have relevant implications in the management of patients.[5,14] **Varices can be classified into small and large by means of a quantitative method, with a suggested cutoff diameter of 5 mm. Alternatively, they can be classified into small, medium, and large by means of a morphological semiquantitative assessment (Table 4-2 and Figure 4-2).** Endoscopy may also identify other features predicting the risk of hemorrhage such as the so-called red signs (see Figure 4-2). The combination of size and appearance of varices and Child-Pugh classification has been proposed to estimate the risk of bleeding, with 1-year likelihood of bleeding ranging from

Table 4-2

Endoscopic Classification of Esophageal and Gastric Varices

Type	Size	Diameter	Characteristics
Esophageal			
F1	Small	< 5 mm	Straight, minimally elevated
F2	Medium	> 5 mm	Tortuous, occupying < 1/3 of the lumen
F3	Large		Tortuous, occupying > 1/3 of the lumen
Gastroesophageal			
GEV1		2 to 5 cm	Communicating with EVs, along the gastric lesser curve
GEV2		2 to 3 cm	Along the gastric greater curve and fundus, more tortuous than GEV1
Isolated gastric varices			
IGV1	Small	< 5 mm	Fundal (rule out splenic vein thrombosis); may occur in the absence of EVs
	Medium	5 to 10 mm	
	Large	> 10 mm	
IGV2			In the gastric corpus, antrum, or pylorus
Additional features			**Characteristics**
Red wale marks			Longitudinal red venules resembling whip marks on the variceal surface
Cherry red spots			Red, discrete, flat spots on varices
Hematocystic spots			Red, discrete, raised spots on varices
Diffuse erythema			Diffuse red color of the varix

GEV1 indicates type 1 gastrointestinal varices; GEV2, type 2 gastrointestinal varices; IGV1, type 1 isolated gastric varices; IGV2, type 2 isolated gastric varices

10% in a Child-Pugh class A patient with small varices without red signs to 75% in a Child-Pugh class C patient with large varices and red signs.[16]

Gastric varices (see Table 4-2 and Figure 4-2) are subdivided according to their size, because it is the main determinant of the risk of bleeding. Gastric varices can be classified into varices that are in continuity with EVs (gastroesophageal varices [GEVs]) and isolated gastric varices (IGVs).[11] GEV

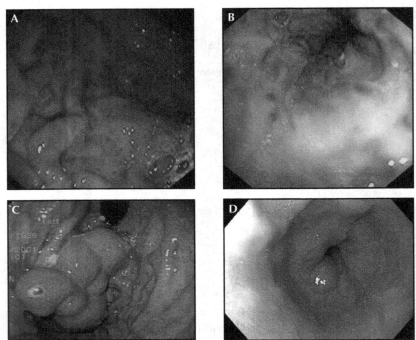

Figure 4-2. Endoscopic characteristics of varices and portal gastropathy. (A) Small EVs. (B) Large EVs with red wale marks (longitudinal red venules resembling whip marks on the variceal surface). (C) Isolated large gastric varix with a hematocystic spot (red, discrete, raised spots on varices). (D) Severe portal hypertensive gastropathy.

are further subdivided into type I GEV (GEV1) and type II GEV (GEV2).[11] GEV1 represent more than 70% of gastric varices, although only 10% ever bleed. IGV are classified into type I IGV (IGV1), which represent less than 10% of gastric varices but tend to bleed more frequently (80%) and, due to their pathophysiological mechanism of formation, are associated with more severe bleeding and a higher rate of hepatic encephalopathy after the bleeding episode, and type II IGV (IGV2), which can be located in the body, antrum, and pylorus.[11] As for EVs, a prognostic index able to predict the likelihood of bleeding from IGV1 has been developed, including Child-Pugh class (risk: C > B > A), variceal size (risk: < 5 mm, 5 to 10 mm, > 10 mm), and presence of red marks (risk: present > absent) combined into a score.

Portal hypertensive gastropathy (see Figure 4-2) refers to a mosaic-like appearance of the gastric mucosa that can be prevalently seen in the fundus and body and less frequently in the antrum of patients with cirrhosis and portal hypertension.[17] From the practical point of view, mild portal hypertensive gastropathy is represented by fine pink speckling of the mucosa, and severe portal hypertensive gastropathy may include cherry red spots that can extend beyond the margins of the reticular network.[18] The reported risk of bleeding from portal hypertensive gastropathy is 3.5% to 31% and 38% to 62% in mild and severe cases, respectively.[11-13] However, acute bleeding from portal hypertensive gastropathy is uncommon, and the most frequent clinical manifestation is chronic blood loss.

Gastric antral vascular ectasia (GAVE) describes the findings of red stripes, separated by normal mucosa, that can be observed in the gastric antrum of patients with various autoimmune diseases, liver cirrhosis, and renal failure. GAVE has also been termed *watermelon stomach* due to its characteristic endoscopic appearance.[19] The occurrence of GAVE is not specific to patients with cirrhosis and portal hypertension, and the pathogenetic mechanisms leading to GAVE development are poorly understood. Although the presence of GAVE is associated with intermittent bleeding, in patients with chronic liver disease **GAVE should be considered an entity distinct from severe portal hypertensive gastropathy.[20] This has a relevant clinical reflex in that GAVE usually does not respond to drugs aimed at lowering portal pressure and does not resolve with placement of a transjugular intrahepatic portosystemic shunt (TIPS).[20,21]**

PREVENTION OF ESOPHAGEAL VARICEAL BLEEDING

Table 4-3 summarizes the clinical applications of measures aimed at prevention of first variceal hemorrhage.

Mechanisms of Action of Drugs Used for the Prevention of Variceal Bleeding

Nonselective β-adrenergic antagonists reduce portal pressure through a reduction of portal blood inflow which is obtained by (1) β_1-adrenergic blockade that decreases the pathologically increased cardiac output, which is typical of the hyperdynamic circulation of cirrhotics; and (2) β_2-adrenergic blockade that indirectly induces vasoconstriction of the splanchnic arteriolar vasculature through unopposed α-adrenergic activity.[22,23] In patients with cirrhosis and no previous bleeding, long-term administration of nonselective β-blockers achieves a reduction in HVPG ≤ 12 mm Hg or a reduction $\geq 20\%$ compared to baseline in 11% and 30% of subjects. These patients are defined as "responders" and can be considered virtually protected from variceal bleeding.[24]

Isosorbide-5-mononitrate is a long-acting nitrate that decreases portal pressure by decreasing postsinusoidal and porto-collateral resistance and indirectly by causing reflex splanchnic vasoconstriction due to decreased cardiac

Table 4-3

Clinical Application of Measures Aimed at Prevention of First Variceal Bleeding

Varices	Additional Features	Management	Recommendations	End-Point
Absent	Any	No treatment	Surveillance every 3 years in compensated patients and annually in the setting of decompensation	Appearance of varices
Small	Compensated disease, no variceal red signs	Nonselective β-blockers (propranolol, nadolol) can be used	Patients who do not receive or do not tolerate β-blockers: surveillance endoscopy every 2 years and at decompensation	Prevention of variceal growth, bleeding, and bleeding-related mortality
	Decompensated disease or variceal red signs	Nonselective β-blockers (propranolol, nadolol) should be used	Patients who do not receive or do not tolerate β-blockers: surveillance endoscopy every year	
Medium/ large	Any	Nonselective β-blockers (propranolol, nadolol)	Titrate drugs to achieve a resting heart rate of 55 bpm or a decrease > 25% compared to baseline; if available, HVPG can be measured to evaluate hemodynamic response; no need for follow-up endoscopy	Prevention of variceal bleeding and bleeding-related mortality
	Patients with contraindications to or who cannot tolerate β-blockers	Endoscopic variceal ligation	Repeat endoscopy every 6 months to identify reappearance of varices	
	Hemodynamic nonresponders			

bmp indicates beats per minute; HVPG, hepatic venous pressure gradient output and arterial vasodilation. The decrease in portal pressure determined by isosorbide-5-mononitrate is mediated by activation of nitric oxide pathways and the occurrence of vasodilation in target vascular beds. Furthermore, a diminished venous return determines a decrease in cardiac output with the occurrence of hypotension and reflex splanchnic vasoconstriction.[25] Acute administration of isosorbide-5-mononitrate may determine a decrease in HVPG of up to 30% to 40%, although tachyphylaxis may occur during chronic administration, and the effects on portal pressure in the individual are not predictable.[23,25,26]

Preprimary Prophylaxis

The only randomized study performed on this topic showed that, in compensated cirrhotic patients without varices and an HVPG > 5 mm Hg, chronic timolol administration was not associated with a significant reduction in development of varices or variceal bleeding after more than 2 years of follow-up, although a post hoc analysis of this study showed that subjects who achieved at least a ≥ 10% reduction in HVPG after 1 year had a significantly lower rate of varices development.[8]

Practical recommendations: Although from the theoretical point of view prevention of varices formation would definitely avoid the risk of bleeding, currently there is no evidence to recommend preprimary prophylaxis for the formation of varices with nonselective β-blockers or any other drug.[14,15]

Primary Prophylaxis in Patients With Small Esophageal Varices

Cirrhotic patients with small EVs have a lower risk of bleeding compared to patients with large varices (about 7% versus 15% at 2-year follow-up), although this difference is balanced when patients with small varices have advanced cirrhosis (Child-Pugh class C) or show endoscopic signs predictive of bleeding (red wale marks).[10,16] Two studies evaluated the use of nonselective β-blockers in this setting and provided contrasting results.[27,28] In the first study, carried out in a mixed population of patients without and with small varices, patients who were randomized to receive propranolol at a fixed dose had a greater risk of developing large varices compared to patients who received placebo (31% versus 14%) after 2-year follow-up,[27] whereas in the second study patients with small varices and low risk of bleeding (no advanced disease and variceal red signs) randomized to receive nadolol titrated according to heart rate had a lower 2-year (7% versus 20%) and 5-year (31% versus 51%) cumulative risk of growth of varices compared to placebo.[28] The use of nonselective β-blockers in cirrhotic patients also seems to be associated with a decreased incidence of other complications such as spontaneous bacterial peritonitis, ascites, and hepatic encephalopathy,[29] in clinical practice physicians are still reluctant to start primary prophylaxis in patients with small varices.

Practical recommendations: Due to the lack of solid evidence supporting universal treatment with nonselective β-blockers in all patients with small varices, it is suggested that nonselective β-blockers should be used for the prevention of growth in size and bleeding of varices in cirrhotic patients with small varices and a high risk of bleeding (ie, decompensated disease, presence of red signs on varices), and patients with compensated cirrhosis and small varices without red signs can be treated with this class of drugs. In patients who receive β-blockers prophylaxis it is not necessary to perform follow-up endoscopy.[14,15]

Primary Prophylaxis in Patients With Medium/Large Esophageal Varices

The aim of treatment in patients with medium/large varices is to reduce bleeding and bleeding-related mortality rates. This can be accomplished with the use of nonselective β-blockers and endoscopic variceal band ligation (EBL). Whether EBL should be preferred to pharmacologic therapy is still a matter of debate.[30] The results of meta-analyses comparing these 2 treatments have shown a benefit using EBL in preventing bleeding compared to pharmacologic therapy, although this difference disappears when larger studies with longer follow-up alone are taken into account. No difference in mortality rates has been demonstrated between these 2 prophylactic treatments.[31,32]

Nonselective β-Blockers

Use of nonselective β-blockers (propranolol, nadolol) is associated with a 45% decrease in the risk of first variceal bleeding and 50% decrease in the risk of bleeding-related death compared to placebo.[10] Factors associated with treatment failure include younger age, large varices, advanced liver disease, and lower dose of β-blocker, and good compliance with treatment is associated with better outcome. A decrease in HVPG < 12 mm Hg or a decrease > 20% with respect to the baseline value has been identified as the most important predictor of protection from bleeding and decreased bleeding-related mortality.[4,10] When treatment with β-blockers is discontinued, the likelihood of bleeding is similar to that of untreated patients.[33]

Isosorbide-5-Mononitrate With or Without Nonselective β-Blockers

Use of isosorbide-5-mononitrate alone is associated with a nonsignificant tendency to increased bleeding and mortality rates compared to propranolol, and its long-term administration has resulted in increased mortality in patients > 50 years.[10,34,35] In patients who cannot tolerate β-blockers, the bleeding rates with isosorbide-5-mononitrate alone are similar to placebo.[36]

Combination therapy with nonselective β-blockers plus isosorbide-5-mononitrate is associated with a nonsignificant decrease in bleeding rate, a similar bleeding-related mortality rate, and a greater incidence of treatment-related side effects compared to β-blockers alone,[37,38] although bleeding rate in patients with large varices alone is not significantly decreased (propranolol, 17% versus propranolol plus isosorbide-5-mononitrate, 20%).[39] Thus, current guidelines do not suggest the use of either isosorbide-5-mononitrate alone or isosorbide-5-mononitrate with nonselective β-blockers for primary prophylaxis of variceal bleeding.

Endoscopic Variceal Band Ligation

EBL determines a mechanic obliteration of the varices and obstruction to the variceal blood flow. The bands are applied starting from the gastroesophageal junction and proceeding upward. Five to 10 bands are applied in each session. Ligation sessions can be repeated every 2 to 3 weeks until complete varices eradication, although there is evidence that increasing the interval between sessions to 8 weeks does not decrease the success rate and has fewer side effects.[40] Follow-up endoscopy should be performed after 6 months, 1 year, and then annually in order to identify reappearance of varices.

The prophylactic use of EBL as compared to no active treatment leads to a significant reduction in bleeding (relative risk decrease = 64%) and mortality rates.[41] There is a small but significant advantage of EBL compared to nonselective β-blockers in terms of incidence of first variceal hemorrhage with no difference on mortality, and patients on nonselective β-blockers tend to have more side effects (13% versus 4%), although side effects are more severe with EBL (including bleeding and bleeding-related death).[42] Although prophylactic EBL seems to be more efficacious compared to β-blockers in the short term, the financial costs of the endoscopic procedure are higher, recurrence of varices can be as high as 60% at 1 year, and its efficacy has not been evaluated in the long term.[22,31,42] Thus, clinical guidelines currently suggest that either EBL or nonselective β-blockers can be used for the prophylaxis of first bleeding in patients with medium/large varices and a high risk of bleeding (ie, decompensated disease, presence of red signs on varices), whereas nonselective β-blockers are the first option in patients without these risk factors and EBL should be reserved for patients who have contraindication or are intolerant to nonselective β-blockers.[14,15] On clinical grounds, due to the subtle and inconsistent differences in efficacy of the 2 treatment modalities, choice of either treatment is more frequently based on patient characteristics, local resources, and expertise.

Practical Recommendations

Nonselective β-blockers (ie, nadolol, propranolol) and EBL are the only treatments that can be used for the prevention of first variceal bleeding in patients with medium or large varices who have never bled. Nonselective β-blockers are the preferred choice in patients who are not at increased risk of bleeding (ie, compensated disease, absence of red sings on varices). In patients with increased risk of bleeding (ie, decompensated disease, presence of red signs on

varices), either prophylactic EBL or nonselective β-blockers can be used. Furthermore, EBL should be performed in patients who have contraindications or are intolerant to nonselective β-blockers and may be preferred as the first prophylactic option in centers with particular endoscopic expertise and/or where patients on pharmacologic therapy cannot be adequately monitored.[14,15]

Guide to Selection and Administration of Nonselective β-Blockers

Propranolol and nadolol are the 2 nonselective β-blockers that are commonly used for both variceal bleeding and rebleeding prophylaxis in cirrhotic patients. Both drugs are inexpensive and can be administered orally. Nadolol has the advantage of being administered once daily due to its prolonged half-life, and because it does not cross the blood-brain barrier it has a lower likelihood of causing central side effects. Absolute (severe chronic obstructive pulmonary disease, congestive heart failure, severe aortic valve stenosis, second- and third-degree atrio-ventricular heart block, peripheral arterial disease) and relative contraindications (insulin-dependent diabetes mellitus, sinus bradycardia, arterial hypotension) are present in 5% to 20% of patients and may limit their use. They should be started at a low dose (ie, 20 mg twice daily for propranolol, 40 mg once daily for nadolol) and should be increased stepwise, while monitoring blood pressure and heart rate until a resting heart rate of 55 beats per minute is reached or a 25% reduction in heart rate compared to baseline. Some patients reaching these targets will be protected from variceal bleeding, although there is no direct correlation between the degree of resting heart rate reduction and decrease in HVPG. Ideally, the best way to assess individual response to pharmacologic prophylaxis would be measurement of HVPG, with patients achieving an HVPG < 12 mm Hg or a reduction > 20% compared to baseline identified as responders and protected from bleeding. However, HVPG measurement is invasive, expensive, and not available in many centers. Furthermore, because there is evidence that at least 60% of patients on β-blocker primary prophylaxis and not achieving these HVPG targets will not bleed during a 2-year follow-up, the use of HVPG for monitoring pharmacologic response to primary prophylaxis is questionable.[43] The maximum dose is 120 mg twice daily for propranolol and 160 mg once daily for nadolol, although the majority of patients usually cannot tolerate these doses due to development of symptoms. Side effects of treatment (severe fatigue, severe bradycardia, symptomatic hypotension, shortness of breath, impotence) develop in 15% to 20% of treated patients and are a cause of dose reduction or treatment withdrawal. **If a patient cannot tolerate propranolol, he or she can be switched to nadolol, and vice versa,**

because sometimes side effects may become less severe. Upon drug discontinuation, the risk of bleeding is similar to pretreatment, and patients should be instructed not to withdraw treatment abruptly due to the risk of rebound bleeding.

MANAGEMENT OF ACUTE ESOPHAGEAL VARICEAL BLEEDING

In cirrhotic patients, ruptured EVs account for approximately 70% of all upper digestive bleeding episodes and are the second most common cause of death.[44] The annual incidence rate of first variceal bleeding in untreated patients ranges from approximately 2% in patients with no varices to 5% in those with small varices and up to 15% in patients with medium to large varices. Other predictors of bleeding are the presence of advanced liver disease (Child-Pugh class C) and red wale marks at endoscopy.[10,16] Despite increased application of prophylaxis and advances achieved in the treatment of hemorrhage, a bleeding episode still carries a mortality rate of up to 20% within 6 weeks.[45] Independent factors associated with continuous bleeding, failure of first-line treatment, and poorer prognosis are advanced Child-Pugh class, an HVPG > 20 mm Hg, and active bleeding at endoscopy. The causes of death after a variceal bleeding episode are mainly uncontrolled bleeding, early rebleeding, sepsis, and renal failure.[46]

Clinical Presentation and Management

Variceal bleeding usually presents with hematemesis and/or melena in a patient with known liver disease, although it can be the first manifestation of cirrhosis in a patient not aware of having chronic liver disease. Patients with suspected acute variceal bleeding should be managed in an intensive care unit, possibly with a multidisciplinary approach, including an endoscopist, hepatologist, interventional radiologist, and a transplant or hepato-biliary surgeon. In general, the majority of patients are admitted to hospitals that do not have all these specialties, and therefore initial management of patients is dictated by locally available technical skills and expertise. However, management of patients may eventually require transfer to tertiary care centers with availability of all these services. According to a consensus conference statement, an acute variceal bleeding episode can be defined as clinically significant when there is blood transfusion requirement of at least 2 units within a 24-hour period from the time of hospitalization for the bleed (time zero) and a systolic pressure less than 100 mm Hg or a postural drop of 20 mm Hg and/or pulse rate greater than 100 beats per minute at time zero.[5,14]

The goals of early management of a variceal bleeding episode include the following (Table 4-4):

- Measures aimed at hemodynamic resuscitation and airway protection
- Pharmacological and endoscopic hemostatic treatment for control of bleeding and prevention of rebleeding
- Prevention and management of complications

Hemodynamic Resuscitation and Airway Protection

Hemodynamic Resuscitation

Hemodynamic resuscitation should be initiated once the airway has been protected and the blood loss has been estimated. At least 2 large-bore peripheral intravenous catheters must be introduced. In the case of significant blood loss and initial volume depletion, circulation should be sustained by means of gelatin-based colloids or albumin and blood products by intravenous administration. Dextrans, hydroxy-ethyl starch, and Ringer's lactate should be avoided because they have detrimental effects on bleeding times and liver function. Packed red blood cells should be administered in order to avoid overtransfusion, because a rapid increase in circulating volume may lead to rebound increase in portal pressure and facilitate rebleeding. In cirrhotic patients there is a correlation between portal pressure and volemia, and during the correction of hypovolemia portal pressure increases more rapidly than volemia.[47] **Recommendations from consensus conferences suggest maintaining a mean arterial pressure at 80 mm Hg and a hemoglobin level at around 8 to 9 g/dL.**[5,14] There is no consensus on the use of platelet transfusion and fresh frozen plasma to correct hemostatic abnormalities, because there is no evidence that these modalities are able to improve patients' prognosis and adequately correct coagulopathy, whereas they are associated with the risk of volume overload. The use of recombinant factor VII together with endoscopic treatment is associated with improved hemostasis rates compared with endoscopic treatment alone, although it has no effect on patient survival, and therefore its use cannot be routinely recommended.[48,49]

Airway Protection

Aspiration pneumonia, airway obstruction, and hypoxemia induced by hemorrhagic shock are major complications of a variceal bleeding episode and should be carefully avoided because they are associated with a high mortality rate due to multi-organ failure. Airway intubation should be performed in patients with impaired mental status or severe bleeding in order to maintain the integrity of the airway and avoid aspiration. Oxygen therapy must be performed to maintain oxygen saturation over 95%. Subjects who have aspiration pneumonia when hemostasis is achieved after failure of first-line therapy have a higher mortality compared to those without this complication.

Table 4-4

Management of Acute Variceal Bleeding

I. Hemodynamic Resuscitation and Airway Protection

Peripheral large-bore IV catheters Urinary catheter Airway intubation (if altered mental status and/or severe bleeding)	Infuse colloid solutions or albumin Packed red cells Platelets and fresh frozen plasma only if needed Oxygen therapy	Maintain MAP at ~80 mm Hg Maintain urinary output at least 50 cc/hour Maintain hemoglobin level ~8 g/dL Do not "overtransfuse": ↑ risk of rebleeding Keep oxygen saturation at least 95%

II. Control of Bleeding and Prevention of Rebleeding

Start pharmacologic treatment as soon as possible	Terlipressin (1 to 2 mg slow intravenous bolus every 4 hours) Somatostatin (initial intravenous 250 µg bolus followed by 250 µg/hour continuous infusion) Octreotide (initial 50 µg intravenous bolus followed by 25 µg/h continuous infusion)	Continued treatment with vasoactive drugs for at least 5 days Avoid terlipressin in older patients and patients with known CV diseases Check glucose during somatostatin therapy Octreotide has less effect on ↓ HVPG
Perform endoscopy (diagnostic and therapeutic) in a hemodynamically stable patient	Variceal ligation (5 to 10 bands per session) should be preferred, when available, due to improved efficacy and lower side effects Injection sclerotherapy can be performed in the case of severe bleeding with limited vision during endoscopy or when ligation is not available	IV erythromycin administration (250 mg) before endoscopy may help clear the stomach of blood Endoscopy should be better performed after vasoactive drugs to obtain a better vision Use proton pump inhibitors to prevent bleeding from treatment-induced esophageal ulcers

(continued)

Table 4-4
Management of Acute Variceal Bleeding (continued)

III. Prevention and Treatment of Complications		
Infections are common in bleeding patients and are associated with poorer prognosis In ascitic patients, obtain a tap for culture and guide antibiotic treatment	Oral norfloxacin (400 mg bid) is the treatment of choice Intravenous ceftriaxone (2 g/daily) is at least as effective as oral norfloxacin	Antibiotic prophylaxis should be continued for at least 5 days after bleeding
Hepatic encephalopathy may be triggered by bleeding	Lactulose or lactitol can be administered by mouth or by enema	Evaluate other causes responsible for altered mental status (electrolyte disturbances, glucose abnormality, renal failure) Perform EEG and CT/MRI of the head in the case of persistent mental alteration despite adequate treatment
Occurrence of renal failure is associated with poorer prognosis	Fluid and electrolytes should be carefully administered to maintain renal perfusion and avoid extravascular volume expansion Use of terlipressin for the treatment of bleeding may be associated with improved renal perfusion	Avoid overuse of diuretics, vascular contrast mediums, and nephrotoxic drugs (aminoglycosides, NSAIDs)

IV indicates intravenous; MAP, mean arterial pressure; CV, cardiovascular; HVPG, hepatic venous pressure gradient; bid, twice daily; EEG, electroencephalography; CT, computed tomography; MRI, magnetic resonance imaging, NSAIDs, nonsteroidal anti-inflammatory drugs

Control of Bleeding and Prevention of Rebleeding

In the context of active bleeding, the aim of treatment is to control bleeding and prevent rebleeding. The first step of specific measures aimed at control of bleeding is institution of pharmacologic therapy with vasoactive drugs (terlipressin, somatostatin, or analogs), followed by endoscopic treatment (injection sclerotherapy, variceal band ligation). **Current guidelines recommend starting pharmacologic therapy with vasoactive drugs as soon as possible and maintaining it for up to 5 days after admission, because this is the period in which early rebleeding most frequently occurs.[14,15] Furthermore, performance of**

diagnostic and therapeutic endoscopy is facilitated by the previous use of vasoactive drugs, because pharmacologic treatment decreases intravariceal pressure and bleeding. Selection of vasoactive drugs should be driven by local resources and be limited to terlipressin or somatostatin and its synthetic analog octreotide.

Pharmacologic Therapy With Vasoactive Drugs

Terlipressin (triglycyl-lysine-vasopressin) is an inactive, synthetic analog of vasopressin that is activated after the glycyl residue is cleaved. A powerful splanchnic arteriolar vasoconstriction, which decreases the portal blood inflow and therefore portal pressure, is the mechanism of action through which terlipressin is able to control variceal bleeding. Terlipressin can be administered by slow intravenous boluses every 4 hours at a dosage of 1 to 2 mg, depending on body weight, for 5 days. Terlipressin causes systemic vasoconstriction with increased peripheral resistance and reduced cardiac output, heart rate, and coronary blood flow; thus, special attention must be paid to patients with known risk factors for cardiovascular disease.[50] Terlipressin administration achieves a higher rate of hemostasis and is the only drug associated with increased survival compared to placebo.[10,51] Side effects include cardiac ischemia and arrhythmia and extremities ischemia (terlipressin is currently not available in the United States).

Somatostatin is a naturally occurring peptide named for its growth hormone-inhibiting properties. It causes an increase in splanchnic vascular resistance by inhibiting the release of splanchnic vasodilator hormones like glucagon, therefore determining a decrease in portal blood inflow. Somatostatin has a short half-life and is rapidly cleared from the circulation. A bolus of somatostatin decreases the HVPG by 52% at 1 minute, 19% at 3 minutes, and 13% at 5 minutes.[52] The schedule of administration of somatostatin during an acute variceal bleeding episode includes an initial intravenous bolus of 250 µg, followed by continuous infusion at a rate of 250 µg/h, for 2 to 5 days. Somatostatin and endoscopic treatment have a positive effect on hemostasis rate compared to endoscopic treatment alone, although there does not seem to be a significant improvement in survival rate.[46] In cirrhotic patients the effects of somatostatin on portal pressure are variable, and a recent study has shown that a modified schedule of administration with three 250-µg boluses followed by continuous infusion of higher doses of somatostatin (500 µg/h) in patients with active bleeding at endoscopy is associated with improved rates of control of bleeding.[53] Due to its very short half-life (1 to 3 minutes), the vasoactive effect of somatostatin is lost soon after intravenous infusion is discontinued. Side effects associated with somatostatin are rare and include hyperglycemia and abdominal cramps.

Octreotide is a synthetic analog of somatostatin that has a longer duration of action but is associated with a less profound decrease in HVPG compared to somatostatin and has been used in various clinical trials in the management of acute variceal bleeding. Octreotide is given intravenously in a continuous infusion of 25 μg/h for 5 days, preceded by a 50-μg intravenous bolus.

Octreotide, in association with endoscopic treatment, has shown to be significantly more effective than placebo or no treatment in obtaining control of active bleeding and in preventing early rebleeding in clinical trials, although it has no effect on survival.[54]

Endoscopic Therapy

Endoscopic examination is fundamental in order to identify the source of bleeding and obtain hemostasis. Endoscopic treatment of EVs can be carried out by means of injection sclerotherapy or variceal band ligation. The choice of endoscopic treatment depends on local expertise and available resources, although variceal band ligation should be preferred because it has been shown to be associated with fewer complications, lower rates of rebleeding, and lower mortality. Endoscopic injection sclerotherapy can be used in clinical situations in which variceal band ligation is difficult to perform, such as when active hemorrhage limits the field of vision during endoscopy.

Timing of Endoscopy

There is no evidence to suggest that early endoscopy versus delayed endoscopy has a beneficial effect on important clinical outcomes (failure to control bleeding, rebleeding, and survival rate). It is of fundamental importance to perform endoscopy on an adequately prepared and hemodynamically stable patient. However, for patients in whom hemodynamic stability cannot be achieved despite adequate support measures and pharmacologic treatment, early endoscopy should be performed in order to stop active bleeding as hemodynamic instability is an independent predictor of rebleeding and death.

Clearing the Stomach

The quality of endoscopic viewing is essential to identify the source of bleeding and perform endoscopic hemostasis safely. A clearer vision can be obtained by gastric lavages through a nasogastric tube or by intravenous infusion of low-dose erythromycin. Erythromycin infusion clears the stomach, stimulating peristalsis by means of its motilin-agonist pharmacologic properties. **Erythromycin infusion (250 mg) 20 minutes before endoscopy is associated with an improved quality and a shorter duration of endoscopy also in bleeding cirrhotic patients.[55]**

Endoscopic Injection Sclerotherapy

Endoscopic injection sclerotherapy (EIS) is based upon the principle of variceal thrombosis by injection of a sclerosing agent. Injections are directed at the bleeding sites in an acutely bleeding patient. Paravariceal injections are effective in decreasing blood oozing due to parietal edema and varix constriction, and this may facilitate subsequent intravariceal injection of the sclerosant. Injections should be initially performed at the gastroesophageal junction and subsequently in an ascending fashion along the distal 5 cm of the esophagus. Various types of sclerosing agents can be used, although there are no data to decide about an optimal sclerosant agent. Likewise, the volume of sclerosant injected at each site is usually around 1 to 2 mL, although the practice of EIS is still largely empiric and individualized. EIS controls active bleeding from varices in 62% to 100% of patients. Once hemostasis has been achieved with emergency EIS, it can be repeated within 1 week and later at intervals every 1 to 3 weeks until eradication of varices.[44,47] Varices may recur in up to 70% of patients after initial eradication. Thus, after varices eradication, surveillance endoscopy should be performed at 6 months and 1 year and later at annual intervals. EIS is associated with local (esophageal ulceration, stricture formation, organ perforation, mediastinitis) and systemic (sepsis, portal vein thrombosis, pleural effusion) complications, and some can be serious and life-threatening. The most common complications are dysphagia and esophageal ulceration, although bleeding from ulcers is not frequent. Proton pump inhibitors can be used to prevent postsclerotherapy ulcer bleeding.[56]

Endoscopic Variceal Band Ligation

EBL is associated with fewer complications than injection sclerotherapy and, if technically feasible, should be preferred. Because the device at the tip of the endoscope may limit the field of vision during examination, performing EBL in a patient with active bleeding may be difficult. EBL has been compared to EIS in several trials and at least 2 meta-analyses, showing that variceal ligation is superior to sclerotherapy in terms of rebleeding rates and patient survival.[41] Esophageal strictures, bleeding from ligation-induced esophageal ulcers, and systemic complications are less common with endoscopic variceal ligation than with injection sclerotherapy. Mucosal ulceration can be observed in up to 90% of patients 1 week after the procedure.[41] There is evidence that administration of proton pump inhibitors is associated with the formation of significantly smaller ulcers and a lower likelihood of post-banding ulcer bleeding, and therefore their use is advisable to decrease treatment-related morbidity.[56]

Prevention and Management of Complications

Bacterial infection—including spontaneous bacterial peritonitis—sepsis, hepatic encephalopathy, and renal failure complicating a bleeding episode are associated with increased mortality[57,58]; therefore, preventing and treating complications associated with variceal bleeding is of utmost importance.[57,58]

Preventing and Treating Infections

Bacterial infections are documented in 30% to 40% of cirrhotic patients at admission or within the first week after the episode of variceal bleeding.

The most common infections are spontaneous bacterial peritonitis, urinary tract infections, and pneumonia. Generally, infections are caused by enterobacteria, and patients may develop sepsis. Infections can increase the risk of early rebleeding and mortality. Use of antibiotics during a bleeding episode is associated with improved survival,[57] and antibiotic prophylaxis is associated with a diminished need of blood transfusions after endoscopic treatment of variceal bleeding. In patients who already had or develop ascites following hemorrhage, a tap should be obtained, and an ascitic fluid culture must be performed. **Both intravenous ceftriaxone (2 g/daily) and oral norfloxacin (400 mg bid) are effective in preventing infections after variceal bleeding.[57] Antibiotic prophylaxis should be instituted as soon as possible and continued for at least 5 days after bleeding.[14,15]**

Hepatic Encephalopathy

The occurrence of hepatic encephalopathy during a variceal bleeding episode may have several causes. Increased circulating ammonia concentration is derived by blood protein degradation in the intestine and decreased hepatic first-pass metabolism due to portal-systemic shunting. Furthermore, the coexistence of bacterial infections, electrolyte disturbances, serum glucose abnormalities, and renal failure may contribute to precipitating an episode of hepatic encephalopathy. Lastly, sedation may be necessary during airway intubation or endoscopy, and this may alter the mental status of the patient. Treatment of hepatic encephalopathy is based on lactulose or lactitol administration by means of repeated enemas or nasogastric tube once bleeding is controlled. In the case of persistence of an altered mental status despite adequate treatment, an electroencephalogram and a computed tomography (CT) scan or magnetic resonance imaging (MRI) of the head should be performed in order to identify other causes of coma.

Renal Failure

Water retention, decreased urinary sodium output, and low glomerular filtration rate are frequent in patients with cirrhosis, and bleeding can worsen renal dysfunction.[58] A urinary catheter should be placed and urinary output must be monitored. Fluids and electrolytes must be infused to maintain renal perfusion pressure and a urinary output of at least 50 cc/h. Concomitant use of terlipressin (not currently available in the United States) for the treatment of bleeding may be associated with an improvement in renal function due to volume redistribution. **The use of nephrotoxic drugs must be avoided, especially aminoglycoside antibiotics, nonsteroidal anti-inflammatory drugs, and vascular contrast mediums. Excessive diuretics use is discouraged because they can aggravate volume depletion. Occurrence of renal failure and the requirement for renal replacement therapy confers a poor prognosis in patients who are not suitable for liver transplantation.**

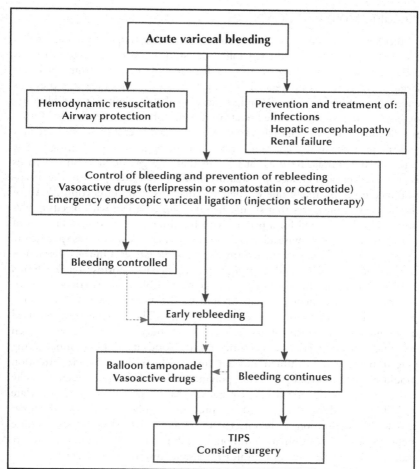

Figure 4-3. Management of an acute variceal bleeding episode.

Practical Recommendations

The first-line treatment of active esophageal variceal hemorrhage is a combination of pharmacologic therapy and endoscopic treatment, which is superior to either modality alone. Terlipressin and somatostatin are the preferred vasoactive drugs, though octreotide can be used if these drugs are not available. EBL should be preferred to EIS due to better outcome and a more favorable adverse effect profile. In the case of severe, active bleeding, EIS can be preferred due to technical ease of sclerotherapy over band ligation in this setting. Figure 4-3 summarizes management of a cirrhotic patient during an acute variceal bleeding episode.

Bleeding From Gastric Varices

Bleeding from gastric varices tends to occur less frequently compared to EVs, although a well-conducted follow-up study reported a 1-year cumulative incidence of bleeding of 16%, a feature not different from medium/large EVs.[60] There is no general agreement upon the relevance that previous endoscopic obliteration of EVs might have on the development and bleeding of gastric varices, because the literature reports contrasting results.[61,62] Other risk factors for bleeding gastric varices are advanced liver disease, variceal size, and the presence of red signs on varices. The management of bleeding gastric varices is not standardized as for EVs, in that intragastric location of varices is also relevant, and endoscopic treatment of EVs reportedly led to the disappearance of GEV, likely due to their peculiar vascular connections.[11] All of the supportive measures that should be taken for a patient with bleeding EVs should also be adopted for a patient with bleeding gastric varices. The use of vasoactive drugs is likewise advisable, although there are no studies specifically reporting their efficacy in the treatment of gastric varices. On the other hand, endoscopic treatment and transjugular intrahepatic portosystemic shunts (TIPS) play a relevant role in the management of bleeding gastric varices. In this case, the treatment of choice should be EIS because in this situation it proved to be safer and more effective than EBL.[63] The obliterating agent used in the injective treatment of gastric varices is N-butyl-2-cyanoacrylate, which is a glue that polymerizes upon contact with blood, developing an occluding plug into the variceal lumen and determining hemostasis. Special attention should be paid to avoid premature polymerization of the glue because it may cause damage to the endoscopic equipment. Mixing N-butyl-2-cyanoacrylate with Lipiodol decreases the risk of premature polymerization and allows radiologic visualization of the injected vessel. Potential risks of this procedure include splenic infarction and pulmonary embolism. TIPS can be used where endoscopic treatment is not technically feasible in refractory cases.[64]

Definition and Management of First-Line Treatment Failure

Approximately 50% of variceal bleeding episodes cease spontaneously, and combined pharmacologic and endoscopic first-line therapy is able to achieve hemostasis in approximately 80% of cases.[65] Nevertheless, a proportion of patients ranging from 10% to 20% do not achieve control of bleeding despite proper management of a variceal bleed.[44]

Definition

The operative definitions contained in Table 4-5 have been suggested by a consensus conference, and although they have been designed with the aim to standardize the nomenclature of clinical trials, their use may help categorize

---
Table 4-5

Operative Definitions of First-Line Treatment Failure

Failure to Control Bleeding
Hematemesis occurring after the first 6 hours along with either a reduction in systolic blood pressure by 20 mm Hg from the 6-hour time point and/or an increase in pulse rate by 20 beats per minute from the 6-hour time point on 2 consecutive readings 1 hour apart or the need for transfusion of 2 or more units of packed red blood cells to increase the hematocrit > 27% or hemoglobin > 9 g/dL.
Rebleeding
Any bleeding that occurs more than 48 hours after the initial admission for variceal hemorrhage and is separated by at least a 24-hour bleeding-free period.
Failure to Prevent Rebleeding
Defined as a single rebleeding episode meeting the criteria for clinically significant bleeding. Rebleeding occurring within 6 weeks of onset of an acute bleeding episode represents early rebleeding; those that occur later are defined as late rebleeding episodes.

patients and select the appropriate management.[14] Risk factors associated with failure to control bleeding include the presence of spurting varices during endoscopy, portal vein thrombosis, a high Child-Pugh score, occurrence of infection, and an elevated HVPG. The risk of early rebleeding following EBL ranges from 8% to 20%, and the risk is greatest within the first 5 days after the initial bleeding episode.[31,44] Early rebleeding after EBL, and less frequently after EIS, may occur from both varices and procedure-associated ulcers. Early rebleeding from varices is strongly associated with increased mortality. Late rebleeding is often associated with large varices, advanced Child-Pugh score, continued alcohol abuse, and the presence of hepatocellular carcinoma.[44]

Management

Patients who fail first-line therapy should be managed in a tertiary care center with availability of adequate radiologic and surgical facilities. Treatment should be aimed at achieving hemostasis, preventing further rebleeding, and improving survival (see Figure 4-3). An attempt at obtaining endoscopic hemostasis can be repeated in patients who present with early rebleeding before proceeding to other measures.[65] Although from the theoretical standpoint orthotopic liver transplantation is the only therapeutic modality that is able to definitively treat failures of first-line treatment, it cannot be acutely performed with this indication alone. Therefore, effective hemostasis should be obtained by other means such as TIPS or portal decompressive surgery. TIPS, in particular, can be used as a salvage bridge to liver transplantation. Temporary balloon tamponade can be used to stop bleeding during the wait for more effective treatment or patient transfer.

■─────────────── Table 4-6 ───────────────■

Contraindications and Complications of TIPS Placement

Contraindications	
Absolute	Severe congestive heart failure
	Severe pulmonary arterial hypertension
	Polycystic liver disease
	Large, hypervascular liver tumors
	Uncontrolled hepatic encephalopathy not related to bleeding
	Portal vein thrombosis with cavernoma
Relative	Portal vein thrombosis without cavernous transformation
	Severe liver failure
	Biliary obstruction
	Active infection (local/systemic)
Complications	
Procedure-related	Neck hematoma
	Liver capsule rupture
	Hemobilia
Stent-related	Thrombosis (early ↓ rate with PTFE-covered stents)
	Stenosis (late)
	Stent migration
	Hemolysis
Portosystemic shunting-related	Hepatic encephalopathy
	Liver failure

TIPS indicates transjugular intrahepatic portosystemic shunt; PTFE, polytetrafluoroethylene

Balloon tamponade with a Sengstaken-Blakemore tube can accomplish hemostasis acutely in most subjects, although its use is burdened with airway compromise and a very high incidence of rebleeding when the balloon is deflated. In this setting, the source of rebleeding can be both varices and damage to the esophageal mucosa caused by prolonged inflation of the balloon. It may be used as a temporary measure until definitive therapy can be instituted in an actively bleeding patient. TIPS creates an artificial communication between the hepatic veins and the portal vein, which is obtained by the angiographic route, and allows portal decompression without the need of general anesthesia and the risks associated with major surgery. Table 4-6 reports contraindications and complications of TIPS placement. The results of several studies using TIPS as a salvage treatment for acute variceal bleeding after failure of first-line therapy have consistently shown that TIPS placement can achieve hemostasis in 90% to 95% of cases.[66] **Thus, TIPS can be used as a salvage treatment when active bleeding continues or early rebleeding occurs following first-line medical and endoscopic treatment (see Figure 4-3). Furthermore, TIPS is particularly indicated in the case of bleeding from gastric varices.** However, the 4-week survival rates after TIPS in these settings can vary from 29% to 75%, mainly due to differences in the general and liver disease-related conditions of the patients.[67] The model for end-stage liver disease (MELD) score can be used to assess prognosis of patients undergoing TIPS. Older age (> 70 years) and a MELD score greater than 15 are associated with poor prognosis in both the short and long term.[68] Hepatic encephalopathy is the most common complication of TIPS, and TIPS placement should be discouraged in patients with uncontrollable hepatic encephalopathy not related to bleeding. Because TIPS creates a sudden communication between a relatively high-pressure zone and the right side of the heart, patients with preexisting severe congestive heart failure should not be considered for TIPS. Hemolytic anemia and stent thrombosis are other common, early complications of TIPS whose incidence can be lowered by the use of polytetrafluoroethylene (PTFE)-covered stents.[69] Liver transplantation should be considered in selected patients after TIPS placement as salvage treatment after failure of first-line therapy for variceal bleeding. In patients who have good liver function (Child-Pugh class A) a surgical portosystemic shunt may be an alternative to TIPS. However, surgery is burdened by a high operative risk and a greater incidence of hepatic encephalopathy.

PREVENTION OF VARICEAL REBLEEDING

Patients who have survived a first episode of variceal bleeding have over a 60% risk of rebleeding within 1 to 2 years of the index episode.[44,70] The mortality rate of each rebleeding episode ranges between 20% and 35%. Treatment to prevent variceal rebleeding should be instituted as soon as possible after the initial bleed has been controlled and the patient is stable. The end-points of treatment in these patients are prevention of rebleeding and rebleeding-associated mortality. Treatments that are currently available for the prevention of variceal rebleeding include pharmacologic therapy, endoscopic therapy, TIPS, and surgical shunting.[71] Though pharmacologic, radiologic, and surgical treatments are aimed at reducing portal pressure below a threshold that is known to be associated with variceal bleeding (ie, 12 mm Hg), endoscopic treatment mechanically reduces the risk of bleeding by obliterating the varices.

Pharmacologic Therapy

Use of nonselective β-blockers for the prevention of rebleeding is associated with a reduction in rebleeding rate from 63% to 42%,[10] and propranolol also reduces rebleeding from portal hypertensive gastropathy (from 65% to 38% at 1 year).[72] Although β-blockers have shown no difference in rebleeding and mortality rates compared to EIS, the former treatment is preferred due to the significantly less frequent and severe side effects. The presence of hepatocellular carcinoma, continued alcohol use, and noncompliance with treatment are factors associated with rebleeding in patients treated with β-blockers. Combination therapy with nonselective β-blockers plus isosorbide-5-mononitrate determines a greater portal-hypotensive effect than β-blockers alone.[37] However, the 2 studies comparing this combination treatment with β-blockers alone have obtained contrasting results.[31] Comparison of β-blockers plus isosorbide-5-mononitrate administration to endoscopic treatment has shown that combination therapy is better than EIS alone, and a meta-analysis of studies comparing combination therapy with EBL has shown that the 2 treatment modalities have no different rebleeding and mortality rates.[31] Addition of isosorbide-5-mononitrate to nonselective β-blockers increases the side effects of treatment. **Due to the lack of a clear advantage using nonselective β-blockers plus isosorbide-5-mononitrate instead of nonselective β-blockers alone and the higher incidence of side effects induced by combination therapy that limits patients compliance to treatment, in clinical practice many physicians prefer administering β-blockers alone.**

Endoscopic Treatment

EIS is effective in reducing both rebleeding and mortality, although it is no better than pharmacologic treatment and is associated with side effects that limit its applicability. EBL determines fewer and less severe complications, with lower rebleeding rates and similar mortality, despite requiring more endoscopic sessions to obliterate varices and being associated with a slightly increased risk of variceal recurrence compared to EIS. Therefore, EBL should be considered the endoscopic procedure of choice for preventing rebleeding. EBL sessions should be repeated at 1- to 2-week intervals until complete variceal eradication (usually 2 to 4 sessions). Due to proven benefits, it is advisable to co-administer proton pump inhibitors to reduce ligation-induced esophageal ulcers bleeding.[57] The rate of recurrence of varices following endoscopic eradication is approximately 50% within 2 years[10,31]; therefore, endoscopic surveillance after 3 months and then every 6 months should be instituted for proper identification and treatment of recurrences.

There is no rationale to combine EIS and EBL, because studies have shown that this combination has no advantage and more side effects than variceal banding alone.[70]

Combined Endoscopic and Pharmacologic Treatment

The rationale for this combination therapy takes into account the different mechanisms of action of the 2 treatments (pathophysiologic and mechanical) and the clinical evidence that pharmacologic therapy might protect patients from rebleeding until obtaining complete endoscopic obliteration. Randomized studies and meta-analyses tend to show lower variceal rebleeding rates with combination therapy compared to either pharmacologic therapy or EBL alone.[73,74] These positive results, however, do not seem to be associated with decreased mortality and bleeding-related mortality rates. Currently, there is no general agreement on whether combination therapy should be preferred over either pharmacologic or endoscopic therapy alone. In fact, though clinical guidelines suggest that combination therapy should be the treatment of choice for preventing variceal rebleeding, a consensus conference statement suggests either pharmacologic or endoscopic therapy alone while waiting for more robust results in favor of combined treatment.[14]

TIPS and Decompressive Surgery

TIPS is superior to both pharmacologic (nonselective β-blockers plus isosorbide-5-mononitrate) and endoscopic treatments for the prevention of rebleeding.[70] Although TIPS is associated with a greater risk of developing hepatic encephalopathy, a recent randomized study has shown that early placement of TIPS in patients at high risk of treatment failure (Child-Pugh class C and Child-Pugh class B patients who have persistent bleeding at endoscopy) is associated with a significant reduction in treatment failure and mortality compared to standard endoscopic and pharmacologic treatment.[75] Decompressive surgery and TIPS show similar rebleeding rates, incidence of hepatic encephalopathy, and mortality risks, although TIPS may be associated with more re-interventions due to shunt dysfunction.[67,68] The use of PTFE-covered stents, which have a significantly lower incidence of occlusion and re-intervention compared to bare stents, is able to overcome these drawbacks.[69] Because of this, TIPS using PTFE-covered stents is considered the best salvage therapy for failures of pharmacologic and endoscopic treatment.

Practical Recommendations

Figure 4-4 depicts an algorithm for the prevention of rebleeding from EVs in cirrhotic patients. All patients surviving a variceal bleeding episode and who have no evidence of hemorrhage for at least 24 hours should receive treatment

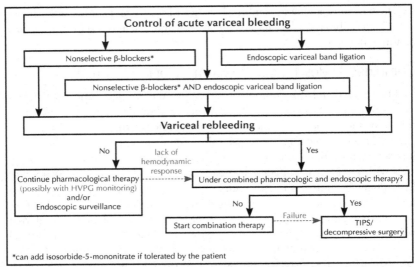

Figure 4-4. Algorithm for the prevention of variceal rebleeding.

aimed at preventing rebleeding. Nonselective β-blockers plus isosorbide-5-mo-nonitrate and EBL alone have similar efficacy. β-blockers should be titrated to the maximum tolerated dose, starting at a low dosage (eg, nadolol 40 mg/daily, propranolol 40 mg twice daily), and if isosorbide-5-mononitrate is considered, then it should be started at 10 mg twice daily and increased to 20 mg twice daily, if tolerated. Pharmacologic therapy has the advantage of being cheap and not requiring surveillance endoscopy. However, few patients can tolerate adequate dosage of dual pharmacologic therapy, and therefore endoscopic treatment alone can be selected in cases of contraindications or intolerance to pharmacologic treatment. **There is increasing evidence that a combination of nonselective β-blockers and EBL should be the treatment of choice, because this treatment seems to be more effective than either treatment alone.**

If rebleeding does not occur, then the patient must continue pharmacologic therapy. The dose of β-blockers should be titrated with the goal of obtaining a heart rate of 55 to 60 beats per minute or a decrease > 25% compared to base-line. Where available, HVPG measurement represents the gold standard for assessing response to pharmacologic therapy, in order to identify hemodynamic nonresponders and implement treatment accordingly. If rebleeding occurs and the patient is not on combined pharmacologic and endoscopic therapy, then this should be initiated. On the other hand, if rebleeding occurs while the patient is on combined therapy, then TIPS with the use PTFE-covered stents should be placed. Currently, radiologic treatment is preferred to decompressive surgery due to similar rates of rebleeding, hepatic encephalopathy, and mortality but with fewer risks. Lastly, patients who have no contraindications should be evaluated for liver transplantation, and in this case the use of TIPS offers several advantages, because a previous decompressive surgical intervention may technically complicate liver transplantation.

REFERENCES

1. D'Amico G, Garcia-Tsao G, Pagliaro L. Natural history and prognostic indicators of survival in cirrhosis: a systematic review of 118 studies. *J Hepatol.* 2006;44:217-231.

2. Chalasani N, Kahi C, Francois F, et al. Improved patient survival after acute variceal bleeding: a multicenter, cohort study. *Am J Gastroenterol.* 2003;98:653-659.

3. Bosch J, Abraldes JG, Berzigotti A, García-Pagan JC. The clinical use of HVPG measurement in chronic liver disease. *Nat Rev Gastroenterol Hepatol.* 2009;6:573-582.

4. Garcia-Tsao G, Groszmann R, Fisher R, Conn HO, Atterbury CE, Glickman M. Portal pressure, presence of gastroesophageal varices and variceal bleeding. *Hepatology.* 1985;5:419-424.

5. de Franchis R. Updating consensus in portal hypertension: report of the Baveno III consensus workshop on definitions, methodology and therapeutic strategies in portal hypertension. *J Hepatol.* 2000;33:846-852.

6. Giannini E, Botta F, Borro P, et al. Platelet count spleen/diameter ratio: proposal and validation of a non-invasive parameter to predict the presence of oesophageal varices in patients with liver cirrhosis. *Gut.* 2003;52:1200-1205.

7. Merli M, Nicolini G, Angeloni S, et al. Incidence and natural history of small esophageal varices in cirrhotic patients. *J Hepatol.* 2003;38:266-272.

8. Groszmann RJ, Garcia-Tsao G, Bosch J, and the Portal Hypertension Collaborative Group. Betablockers to prevent gastroesophageal varices in patients with cirrhosis. *N Engl J Med.* 2005;353:2254-2261.

9. de Franchis R. Non-invasive (and minimally invasive) diagnosis of oesophageal varices. *J Hepatol.* 2008;49:520-527.

10. D'Amico G, Pagliaro L, Bosch J. Pharmacological treatment of portal hypertension: an evidence-based approach. *Semin Liver Dis.* 1999;19:475-505.

11. Sarin SK, Lahoti D, Saxena SP, Murthy NS, Makwana UK. Prevalence, classification, and natural history of gastric varices: a long-term follow-up study in 568 portal hypertension patients. *Hepatology.* 1992;16:1343-1349.

12. Thuluvath PJ, Yoo HY. Portal hypertensive gastropathy. *Am J Gastroenterol.* 2002;97:2973-2978.

13. Merli M, Nicolini G, Angeloni S, Gentili F, Attili AF, Riggio O. The natural history of portal hypertensive gastropathy in patients with liver cirrhosis and mild portal hypertension. *Am J Gastroenterol.* 2004;99:1959-1965.

14. de Franchis R. Evolving Consensus in Portal Hypertension Report of the Baveno IV Consensus Workshop on methodology of diagnosis and therapy in portal hypertension. *J Hepatol.* 2005;43:167-176.

15. Garcia-Tsao G, Sanyal A, Grace ND, Carey W, Practice Guidelines Committee of the American Association for the Study of Liver Diseases, and Practice Parameters Committee of the American College of Gastroenterology. Prevention and management of gastroesophageal varices and variceal hemorrhage in cirrhosis. *Hepatology.* 2007;46:922-938.

16. North Italian Endoscopic Club for the Study and Treatment of Esophageal Varices. Prediction of the first variceal hemorrhage in patients with cirrhosis of the liver and esophageal varices. A prospective multicenter study. *N Engl J Med.* 1988;319:983-989.

17. Spina GP, Arcidiacono R, Bosch J, et al. Gastric endoscopic features in portal hypertension: final report of a consensus conference, Milan, Italy, September 19, 1992. *J Hepatol.* 1994;21:461-467.

18. McCormack TT, Sims J, Eyre-Brook I, et al. Gastric lesions in portal hypertension: inflammatory gastritis or congestive gastropathy? *Gut.* 1985;26:1226-1232.

19. Gostout CJ, Viggiano TR, Ahlquist DA, Wang KK, Larson MV, Balm R. The clinical and endoscopic spectrum of the watermelon stomach. *J Clin Gastroenterol.* 1992;15:256-263.

20. Payen JL, Calès P, Voigt JJ, et al. Severe portal hypertensive gastropathy and antral vascular ectasia are distinct entities in patients with cirrhosis. *Gastroenterology.* 1995;108:138-144.

21. Burak KW, Lee SS, Beck PL. Portal hypertensive gastropathy and gastric antral vascular ectasia (GAVE) syndrome. *Gut.* 2001;49:866-872.

22. Tiani C, Abraldes JG, Bosch J. Portal hypertension: pre-primary and primary prophylaxis of variceal bleeding. *Dig Liver Dis.* 2008;40:318-327.

23. Tripathi D, Hayes PC. Review article: a drug therapy for the prevention of variceal haemorrhage. *Aliment Pharmacol Ther.* 2001;15:291-310.

24. D'Amico G, Garcia-Pagan JC, Luca A, Bosch J. HVPG reduction and prevention of variceal bleeding in cirrhosis: a systematic review. *Gastroenterology.* 2006;131:1624.

25. Blei AT, Garcia-Tsao G, Groszmann RJ, et al. Hemodynamic evaluation of isosorbide dinitrate in alcoholic cirrhosis. Pharmacokinetic-hemodynamic interactions. *Gastroenterology.* 1987;93:576-583.

26. Jones AL, Hayes PC. Organic nitrates in portal hypertension. *Am J Gastroenterol.* 1994;89:7-14.

27. Calès P, Oberti F, Payen JL, et al. Lack of effect of propranolol in the prevention of large esophageal varices in patients with cirrhosis: a randomized trial. French-Speaking Club for the Study of Portal Hypertension. *Eur J Gastroenterol Hepatol.* 1999;11:741-745.

28. Merkel C, Marin R, Angeli P, and the Gruppo Triveneto per l'Ipertensione Portale. A placebo-controlled clinical trial of nadolol in the prophylaxis of growth of small esophageal varices in cirrhosis. *Gastroenterology.* 2004;127:476-484.

29. Abraldes JG, Tarantino I, Turnes J, Garcia-Pagan JC, Rodés J, Bosch J. Hemodynamic response to pharmacological treatment of portal hypertension and long-term prognosis of cirrhosis. *Hepatology.* 2003;37:902-908.

30. de Franchis R. Endoscopy critics vs endoscopy enthusiasts for primary prophylaxis of variceal bleeding. *Hepatology.* 2006;43:24-26.

31. Garcia-Pagan JC, De Gottardi A, Bosch J. Review article: the modern management of portal hypertension—primary and secondary prophylaxis of variceal bleeding in cirrhotic patients. *Aliment Pharmacol Ther.* 2008;28:178-186.

32. Bosch J, Garcia-Tsao G. Pharmacological versus endoscopic therapy in the prevention of variceal hemorrhage: and the winner is.... *Hepatology.* 2009;50;674-677.

33. Talwalkar JA, Kamath PS. An evidence-based medicine approach to beta-blocker therapy in patients with cirrhosis. *Am J Med.* 2004;116:759-766.

34. Angelico M, Carli L, Piat C, Gentile S, Capocaccia L. Isosorbide-5-mononitrate compared with propranolol on first bleeding and long-term survival in cirrhosis. *Gastroenterology.* 1997;113:1632-1639.

35. Garcia-Pagan JC. Non-selective beta-blockers in the prevention of first variceal bleeding. Is there any definite alternative? *J Hepatol.* 2002;37:393-395.

36. Garcia-Pagan JC, Villanueva C, Vila MC, and the MOVE Group. Isosorbide-5-mononitrate in the prevention of the first variceal bleed in patients who cannot receive beta-blockers. *Gastroenterology.* 2001;121:908-914.

37. Garcia-Pagan JC, Feu F, Bosch J, Rodes J. Propranolol compared with propranolol plus isosrbide-5-monitrate for portal hypertension in cirrhosis. A randomized controlled study. *Ann Intern Med.* 1991;114:869-873.

38. Albillos A. Preventing first variceal hemorrhage in cirrhosis. *J Clin Gastroenterol.* 2007;41(suppl 3):S305-S311.

39. García-Pagán JC, Morillas R, Bañares R, and the Spanish Variceal Bleeding Study Group. Propranolol plus placebo versus propranolol plus isosorbide-5-mononitrate in the prevention of first variceal bleed: a double-blind RCT. *Hepatology.* 2003;37:1260-1266.

40. Yoshida H, Mamada Y, Taniai N, et al. A randomized control trial of bi-monthly versus bi-weekly endoscopic variceal ligation of esophageal varices. *Am J Gastroenterol.* 2005;100:2005-2009.

41. Garcia-Pagan JC, Bosch J. Endoscopic band ligation in the treatment of portal hypertension. *Nat Clin Pract Gastroenterol Hepatol.* 2005;2:526-535.

42. Khuroo MS, Khuroo NS, Farahat KL, Khuroo YS, Sofi AA, Dahab ST. Meta-analysis: endoscopic variceal ligation for primary prophylaxis of oesophageal variceal bleeding. *Aliment Pharmacol Ther.* 2005;21:347-361.

43. de Franchis R, Dell'Era A, Iannuzzi F. Acute variceal bleeding: pharmacological treatment and primary/secondary prophylaxis. *Best Pract Res Clin Gastroenterol.* 2008;22:279-294.

44. Habib A, Sanyal AJ. Acute variceal hemorrhage. *Gastrointest Endoscopy Clin N Am.* 2007;17:223-252.

45. Jamal MM, Samarasena JB, Hashemzadeh M. Decreasing in-hospital mortality for oesophageal variceal hemorrhage in the USA. *Eur J Gastroenterol Hepatol.* 2008;20:947-955.

46. Thabut D, Bernard-Chabert B. Management of acute bleeding from portal hypertension. *Best Pract Res Clin Gastroenterol.* 2007;21:19-29.

47. Kravetz D, Sikuler E, Groszmann RJ. Splanchnic and systemic hemodynamics in portal hypertensive rats during hemorrhage and blood volume restitution. *Gastroenterology.* 1986;90(pt 1):1232-1240.

48. Bosch J, Thabut D, Bendtsen F, and the European Study Group on rFVIIa in UGI Haemorrhage. Recombinant factor VIIa for upper gastrointestinal bleeding in patients with cirrhosis: a randomized, double-blind trial. *Gastroenterology.* 2004;127:1123-1130.

49. Bosch J, Thabut D, Albillos A, and the International Study Group on rFVIIa in UGI Hemorrhage. Recombinant factor VIIa for variceal bleeding in patients with advanced cirrhosis: a randomized, controlled trial. *Hepatology.* 2008;47:1604-1614.

50. Villanueva C, Balanzó J. Variceal bleeding: pharmacological treatment and prophylactic strategies. *Drugs.* 2008;68:2303-2324.

51. Ioannou GN, Doust J, Rockey DC. Systematic review: terlipressin in acute oesophageal variceal haemorrhage. *Aliment Pharmacol Ther.* 2003;17:53-64.

52. Cirera I, Feu F, Luca A, et al. Effects of bolus injections and continuous infusions of somatostatin and placebo in patients with cirrhosis: a double-blind hemodynamic investigation. *Hepatology.* 1995;22:106-111.

53. Moitinho E, Planas R, Bañares R, and the Variceal Bleeding Study Group. Multicenter randomized controlled trial comparing different schedules of somatostatin in the treatment of acute variceal bleeding. *J Hepatol.* 2001;35:712-718.

54. Corley DA, Cello JP, Adkisson W, Ko WF, Kerlikowske K. Octreotide for acute esophageal variceal bleeding: a meta-analysis. *Gastroenterology.* 2001;120:946-954.

55. Frossard JL, Spahr L, Queneau PE, et al. Erythromycin intravenous bolus infusion in acute upper gastrointestinal bleeding: a randomized, controlled, double-blind trial. *Gastroenterology.* 2002;123:17-23.

56. Shaheen NJ, Stuart E, Schmitz SM, et al. Pantoprazole reduces the size of postbanding ulcers after variceal band ligation: a randomized, controlled trial. *Hepatology.* 2005;41:588-594.

57. Bernard B, Grangé JD, Khac EN, Amiot X, Opolon P, Poynard T. Antibiotic prophylaxis for the prevention of bacterial infections in cirrhotic patients with gastrointestinal bleeding: a meta-analysis. *Hepatology.* 1999;29:1655-1661.

58. Cárdenas A, Ginès P, Uriz J, et al. Renal failure after upper gastrointestinal bleeding in cirrhosis: incidence, clinical course, predictive factors, and short-term prognosis. *Hepatology.* 2001;34(pt 1):671-676.

59. Bendtsen F, Krag A, Moller S. Treatment of acute variceal bleeding. *Dig Liver Dis.* 2008;40:328-336.

60. Kim T, Shijo H, Kokawa H, et al. Risk factors for hemorrhage from gastric fundal varices. *Hepatology.* 1997;25:307-312.

61. Schepke M, Biecker E, Appenrodt B, Heller J, Sauerbruch T. Coexisting gastric varices should not preclude prophylactic ligation of large esophageal varices in cirrhosis. *Digestion.* 2009;80:165-169.

62. Sarin SK, Shahi HM, Jain M, Jain AK, Issar SK, Murthy NS. The natural history of portal hypertensive gastropathy: influence of variceal eradication. *Am J Gastroenterol.* 2000;95:2888-2893.

63. Lo GH, Lai KH, Cheng JS, Chen MH, Chiang HT. A prospective, randomized trial of butyl cyanoacrylate injection versus band ligation in the management of bleeding gastric varices. *Hepatology.* 2001;33:1060-1064.

64. Ryan BM, Stockbrugger RW, Ryan JM. A pathophysiologic, gastroenterologic, and radiologic approach to the management of gastric varices. *Gastroenterology.* 2004;126:1175-1189.

65. Cheung J, Zeman M, van Zanten SV, Tandon P. Systematic review: secondary prevention with band ligation, pharmacotherapy or combination therapy after bleeding from oesophageal varices. *Aliment Pharmacol Ther.* 2009;30:577-588.

66. Escorsell A, Bañares R, García-Pagán JC, et al. TIPS versus drug therapy in preventing variceal rebleeding in advanced cirrhosis: a randomized controlled trial. *Hepatology.* 2002;35:385-392.

67. Zheng M, Chen Y, Bai J, et al. Transjugular intrahepatic portosystemic shunt versus endoscopic therapy in the secondary prophylaxis of variceal rebleeding in cirrhotic patients: meta-analysis update. *J Clin Gastroenterol.* 2008;42:507-516.

68. Rosado B, Kamath PS. Transjugular intrahepatic portosystemic shunts: an update. *Liver Transpl.* 2003;9:207-217.

69. Bureau C, Garcia-Pagan JC, Otal P, et al. Improved clinical outcome using polytetrafluoroethylene-coated stents for TIPS: results of a randomized study. *Gastroenterology.* 2004;126:469-475.

70. Berzigotti A, García-Pagán JC. Prevention of recurrent variceal bleeding. *Dig Liver Dis.* 2008;40:337-342.

71. Pérez-Ayuso RM, Piqué JM, Bosch J, et al. Propranolol in prevention of recurrent bleeding from severe portal hypertensive gastropathy in cirrhosis. *Lancet.* 1991;337:1431-1434.

72. Gonzalez R, Zamora J, Gomez-Camarero J, Molinero LM, Bañares R, Albillos A. Meta-analysis: combination endoscopic and drug therapy to prevent variceal rebleeding in cirrhosis. *Ann Intern Med.* 2008;149:109-122.

73. Ravipati M, Katragadda S, Swaminathan PD, Molnar J, Zarling E. Pharmacotherapy plus endoscopic intervention is more effective than pharmacotherapy or endoscopy alone in the secondary prevention of esophageal variceal bleeding: a meta-analysis of randomized, controlled trials. *Gastrointest Endosc.* 2009;70:658-664.

74. Kravetz D. Prevention of recurrent esophageal variceal hemorrhage: review and current recommendations. *J Clin Gastroenterol.* 2007;41(suppl 3):S318-S322.

75. Garcia-Pagan JC, Caca K, Bureau C, and the Early TIPS (Transjugular Intrahepatic Portosystemic Shunt) Cooperative Study Group. Early use of TIPS in patients with cirrhosis and variceal bleeding. *N Engl J Med.* 2010;362:2370-2379.

chapter 5

MANAGEMENT OF ASCITES AND RENAL ISSUES IN PATIENTS WITH CIRRHOSIS

Jonathan M. Fenkel, MD and Victor J. Navarro, MD

Ascites is the most common complication of cirrhosis, and 50% of patients with cirrhosis will develop ascites within 10 years of diagnosis.[1] It can usually be managed effectively with a combination of diuretics and salt restriction. Occasionally, other therapies are necessary, which will be discussed in this chapter. **Once ascites develops, it should clue the clinician in to the possibility that a patient may require liver transplantation, because there is an estimated 50% mortality at 2 years from its onset.**[2] Hepatorenal syndrome (HRS) is a discrete form of renal failure occurring in patients with cirrhosis. It complicates 10% of all cirrhotics over their lifetime and is the most common fatal complication of cirrhosis, with less than 50% survival at 2 to 4 weeks.[3,4] This chapter aims to describe the diagnosis and management of both ascites and HRS, as well common associated situations including spontaneous bacterial peritonitis (SBP).

BRIEF PATHOPHYSIOLOGY

Cirrhosis is characterized by intrahepatic vasoconstriction, increased intrahepatic resistance to portal blood flow, and systemic arteriolar vasodilation.[5,6] This results in an overall decrease in systemic vascular resistance, causing a decrease in effective arterial blood volume, which leads to a predictable homeostatic response of renin-angiotensin-aldosterone system (RAAS) activation, sympathetic nervous system activation, and increased release of antidiuretic hormone (ADH). These responses ultimately lead

Zaman A. *Managing the Complications of Cirrhosis: A Practical Approach* (pp 61-76).

━━━━━━━━━━━━━━━━━━ Table 5-1 ━━━━━━━━━━━━━━━━━━

Differential Diagnosis of Ascites

Hepatic Etiology	Nonhepatic Etiology
Cirrhosis	Congestive heart failure
Acute liver failure	Pulmonary hypertension
Alcoholic hepatitis	Nephrotic syndrome
Portal vein thrombosis	Tuberculosis
Budd-Chiari syndrome	Peritoneal carcinomatosis
Massive liver metastasis	Myxedema
Sinusoidal obstruction syndrome (hepatic veno-occlusive disease)	Pancreatitis
	Lymphatic obstruction/leak (chylous ascites)
	Immunologic: C1-esterase inhibitor deficiency, systemic lupus erythematosus

to sodium and water retention and ascites formation. The retention of free water, due to ADH increase, to a greater degree than sodium, leads to dilutional hyponatremia. Additionally, as an early result of the systemic arteriolar vasodilation, heart rate and cardiac output increase in an effort to maintain mean arterial blood pressure. As vasodilation worsens with progression of cirrhosis, the cardiac output is unable to rise further, leading to further activation of the RAAS and sympathetic nervous system, as well as ADH release. These processes, in combination with increased sinusoidal pressures, lead to ascites formation. As this hormonal activation persists, angiotensin, ADH, and the sympathetic nervous system all promote renal vasoconstriction.[5-7] This renal vasoconstriction is the primary mechanism in the development of HRS. The rate at which this vasoconstriction occurs determines whether a patient develops HRS type 1 (rapidly progressive) or type 2 (slowly progressive).[4,8]

DIAGNOSING THE PROBLEM

The majority of patients with ascites have cirrhosis, though approximately 15% will develop ascites of nonhepatic origin.[9] Table 5-1 illustrates the differential diagnosis for ascites.

Ascites is readily diagnosed by physical exam. Flank bulging is the most frequent clinical sign, and percussion of the abdomen reveals shifting dullness if greater than 1.5 L of fluid is present in the abdomen.[1,9] Shifting dullness is

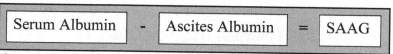

Figure 5-1. Formula for calculation of serum ascites albumin gradient (SAAG).

the most specific physical exam element for ascites and can be performed at the bedside by first percussing the patient in a supine position and noting the line at which the percussion sound changes from dull to tympanitic. Next, ask the patient to rotate onto the side facing you and percuss the abdomen again. The line of percussive change should shift upward with positive shifting dullness. Imaging studies can also be used to diagnose the presence of ascites with high accuracy.[10] Ultrasound, computed tomography (CT), and magnetic resonance imaging (MRI) can all detect the presence of even small quantities of ascitic fluid, including perihepatic ascites. In obese patients, imaging may be necessary because physical examination is more difficult.[1] Once the presence of ascites has been confirmed, abdominal paracentesis should be performed for diagnostic purposes.[1,2] **Ascites from portal hypertension should have a serum-ascites-albumin gradient (SAAG) > 1.1.[1] This simple calculation (Figure 5-1) is helpful in determining whether or not ascites is secondary to portal hypertension. The serum and ascites albumin measurements should be collected on the same day.**

HRS is defined as the presence of renal failure (creatinine > 1.5 mg/dL) in a patient with cirrhosis and ascites without an improvement in creatinine after 48 h of volume expansion with intravenous albumin (1 g/kg/day up to 100 g/day) and withdrawal of diuretics, in the absence of shock, nephrotoxic drugs, and parenchymal renal disease (Table 5-2).[11] Albumin is preferred over saline-based volume expansion in these consensus recommendations.

A urine sodium is not required for diagnosis[4] but is usually < 10, suggesting sodium avidity. The fractional excretion of sodium (FENa) will be less than 1%, making it difficult to distinguish from prerenal azotemia before volume challenge.

HRS is further categorized into type 1 and type 2. Type 1 HRS is a form of acute renal failure, defined by a doubling of the serum creatinine to > 2.5 g/dL in less than 2 weeks.[1,4,8] Type 1 HRS occurs most often in patients with infections, including SBP and gastrointestinal (GI) bleeding. Type 2 HRS has a more indolent course, defined by a slowly progressive increase in serum creatinine in the 1.25 to 2.5 g/dL range over months.[1,4,8] Type 2 HRS occurs most often in patients with refractory ascites.

Other causes of renal failure are also possible in patients with cirrhosis (Table 5-3).

--- Table 5-2 ---

2007 Consensus Diagnostic Criteria for Hepatorenal Syndrome From the International Ascites Club

1. Cirrhosis with ascites
2. Serum creatinine > 1.5 g/dL
3. Absence of improvement in serum creatinine after 2 days of diuretic withdrawal and volume expansion with albumin (1 g albumin/kg/day up to 100 g/day)
4. Absence of shock
5. Absence of recent or current treatment with nephrotoxic medications
6. Absence of parenchymal kidney disease as indicated by proteinuria > 500 mg/ day, microhematuria (> 50 red blood cells/high-power field), and/or abnormal renal ultrasound

Adapted from Salerno F, Gerbes A, Gines P, Wong F, Arroyo V. Diagnosis, prevention and treatment of the hepatorenal syndrome in cirrhosis. *Gut.* 2007;56:1310-1318.

--- Table 5-3 ---

Differential Diagnosis of Renal Failure in Cirrhosis

Hepatorenal syndrome
Prerenal azotemia
Acute tubular necrosis
Parenchymal renal disease
Drug-induced renal failure (aminoglycosides, IV contrast, NSAIDs, etc)
Obstructive renal failure (benign prostatic hypertrophy, prostate cancer, nephrolithiasis)
IV indicates intravenous; NSAIDS, nonsteroidal anti-inflammatory drugs

Prerenal azotemia is often precipitated by gastrointestinal bleeding or overdiuresis. Patients on high doses of lactulose also may develop prerenal azotemia from excessive diarrhea. A fluid challenge helps distinguish between HRS and prerenal azotemia.[4,12] Acute tubular necrosis may also occur in the setting of acute hypovolemia. Urine sediment with tubular epithelial cells favors acute tubular necrosis over HRS, but both may contain granular casts. Hepatitis B is associated with at least 3 types of parenchymal renal disease, including membranous glomerulopathy, membranoproliferative glomerulonephritis, and polyarteritis nodosa-associated vasculitis.[8] Hepatitis C is also associated with various

1. ≥ 250 PMN/mm^3 with a (+) culture for a single organism
2. ≥ 250 PMN/mm^3 with a (−) culture
3. (+) culture for a single organism with < 250 PMN/mm^3

Figure 5-2. Criteria for diagnosis of spontaneous bacterial peritonitis. PMN indicates polymorphonuclear leukocytes.

renal parenchymal diseases, including cryoglobulinemia, membranous glomerulopathy, membranoproliferative glomerulonephritis, and secondary polyarteritis nodosa.[8,12] It is important to exclude these parenchymal diseases before making a diagnosis of HRS. A careful history can help evaluate for drug-induced kidney injury. A renal ultrasound should be ordered to exclude hydronephrosis from any cause leading to obstructive renal failure.

SBP is a high-risk condition for the development of HRS and requires the presence of ascites in order to make the diagnosis.[2] There is a 10% lifetime prevalence of SBP in patients with cirrhosis, but the prevalence of infection approaches 20% to 30% among hospitalized patients with cirrhosis.[2,13] The ascitic fluid in patients with cirrhosis is a protein-deficient environment, where specific protective proteins, including complements, immunoglobulins, and opsonins, are in low concentrations. This makes ascitic fluid particularly susceptible to spontaneous infection. SBP is defined as the presence of bacterial infection in the ascitic fluid, in the absence of another source for infection.[1,2] **SBP can present with fever, abdominal pain, leukocytosis, change in mental status, or sepsis, or it can be asymptomatic up to 20% of the time. Patients with a history of SBP, concomitant GI bleeding, or extremely low protein ascites (fluid total protein < 1 g/dL) are at increased risk of developing SBP.** The diagnosis of SBP is made by performing a paracentesis and measuring the ascitic fluid cell count with differential and fluid culture.[14] There are 3 commonly accepted criteria for SBP diagnosis as listed in Figure 5-2.

An absolute neutrophil count > 250/mm^3 with a positive fluid culture is pathognomic for SBP. However, positive fluid cultures are uncommon, and the diagnosis can be made by cell count alone. The third criteria is also referred to as *nonneutrocytic bacterascites* but is treated as SBP.[2]

ASCITES MANAGEMENT

- Sodium restriction (2 g/day sodium diet = 88 mmol/day).[1-3,13] It is also beneficial for all cirrhotic patients to meet with a nutritionist to help recognize foods that are high in sodium and develop a personalized nutritional plan (Figure 5-3).[9]

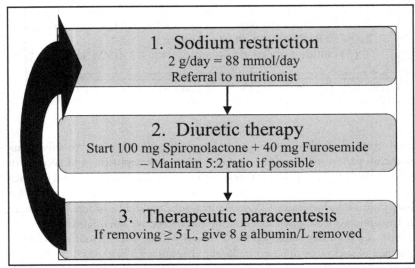

1. Sodium restriction
2 g/day = 88 mmol/day
Referral to nutritionist

2. Diuretic therapy
Start 100 mg Spironolactone + 40 mg Furosemide
– Maintain 5:2 ratio if possible

3. Therapeutic paracentesis
If removing ≥ 5 L, give 8 g albumin/L removed

Figure 5-3. Algorithm for management of uncomplicated ascites. In tense ascites, therapeutic paracentesis should be performed before initiation of diuretic
therapy.

- Diuretics. **The American Association for the Study of Liver
  Disease (AASLD) recommends a combination of spironolactone and furosemide in a 5:2 ratio to maximize diuresis while
  balancing potassium.**[1] **These medications may be increased
  to a maximum of 400 mg spironolactone and 160 mg of
  furosemide.**[1,2] Once daily doses are preferred to split dosing.[1,5] If a
  patient develops painful gynecomastia, amiloride or triamterene may be
  utilized instead of spironolactone.[1,2,13] Limited data on the use of eplerenone exist in cirrhotic patients.[15] **Furosemide monotherapy is not
  recommended because it is inferior to spironolactone alone and
  the combination of spironolactone and furosemide.**[13] If a patient
  develops renal failure while on diuretics, doses may need to be adjusted
  or the medications may need to be discontinued.
- Fluid restriction. **This is <u>not</u> recommended in the management of
  ascites unless the serum sodium is ≤ 125 mmol/L.**[1]
- Therapeutic paracentesis. A large-volume paracentesis should be performed in patients presenting with tense ascites before initiation of
  oral diuretics.[1,9] **Usually up to 5 L can be safely removed without simultaneous albumin infusion. If more than 5 L is to be
  removed, intravenous (IV) albumin should be given at 8 g
  albumin/L fluid removed during the procedure to help prevent**

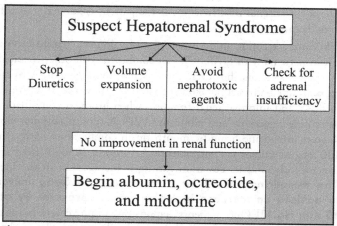

Figure 5-4. Basic approach to the treatment of hepatorenal syndrome.

postparacentesis circulatory dysfunction and incipient hepatorenal syndrome.[1,2,13]

More than 90% of patients with ascites can be effectively managed with a combination of sodium restriction and diuretics alone.[9] Patients with alcoholic liver disease, in particular, can improve synthetic function after cessation of alcohol and may not require long-term diuretics as their abstinence period lengthens.[1,9] Similarly, patients with decompensated hepatitis B cirrhosis can have remarkable improvement on antiviral medication.[1] Patients with underlying parenchymal renal disease may need lower doses of spironolactone to achieve normokalemia.[9]

MANAGEMENT OF HEPATORENAL SYNDROME

- Discontinue diuretics. Any time HRS is suspected, diuretics should be held (Figure 5-4).[1,13]
- Volume expansion. **Given the difficulty in distinguishing HRS from prerenal azotemia, a fluid challenge with IV albumin or 1.5 L of normal saline is the next step.** Most recent reviews favor IV albumin, 1 g/kg/day up to 100 g/day.[5,11] Assessment of intravascular volume status can be difficult in cirrhotic patients with edema and/or ascites, and central venous pressure measurements may be helpful.[4]
- Avoid or discontinue nephrotoxic agents. These agents, including aminoglycosides, nonsteroidal anti-inflammatory drugs, and iodinated contrast, can confound the diagnosis and exacerbate HRS.[4,5,11]

- Check for adrenal insufficiency. If the patient is adrenally insufficient, steroids can improve survival.[4]
- Albumin, octreotide, midodrine. Albumin alone has a mild survival benefit in patients with HRS.[16] When combined with other therapies such as vasoconstrictors, however, there is improved benefit.[1,4] Midodrine, an oral alpha-adrenergic agonist, has been shown to improve survival in HRS and improve renal function when given in combination with octreotide injections and albumin.[1,4,11,16] A typical regimen would be to start midodrine 5 mg by mouth tid in combination with octreotide 100 mcg subcutaneous injections tid.[4] Albumin 20 to 40 g/day is begun concurrently, and its cessation timing is inconsistent in the literature. **The midodrine should be titrated up in 2.5-mg increments to achieve an increase in mean arterial pressure by at least 15 mm Hg.**[4,11] Once patients demonstrate improvement in renal function on this regimen, the albumin can be discontinued and the midodrine and octreotide can be continued on an outpatient basis.[13]

TREATMENT OF SPONTANEOUS BACTERIAL PERITONITIS

- Antibiotics. Treatment of SBP is designed to target the most likely organisms responsible for the infection. If the bacteria is known from culture, antibiotics should be selected to target that specific organism. If the cultures are negative, antibiotics that cover *Escherichia coli, Streptococcus pneumoniae, Klebsiella* species, and some anaerobes are recommended.[17] **First-line therapy is with a third-generation cephalosporin, typically cefotaxime 2 g IV every 8 to 12 h for 5 days.**[1,9,13] Fluoroquinolones and amoxicillin/clavulanate have also been used with good success.[13] Most treatments are 90% effective. If ceftriaxone is chosen, be careful to monitor for new right upper quadrant abdominal pain, because this medication can sometimes precipitate cholelithiasis, microlithiasis, or pseudolithiasis.[18]
- Albumin. **The addition of albumin has been shown to decrease the incidence of HRS and improve mortality in patients with SBP.**[1,8] **It should be dosed 1.5 g/kg on day 1 and 1 g/kg on day 3.** Cost and availability of albumin have hindered widespread use, but it is commonly used in liver transplant centers and is considered the standard of care in acute management of SBP.
- Repeat paracentesis. Most patients do not require repeat paracentesis if they are clinically improved,[1] though some sources recommend a repeat paracentesis after 2 days of treatment to assess for response to therapy.[13,19] Patients on the transplant list are usually made inactive while being treated for SBP, so repeat paracentesis is often performed to document clearance of infection before reactivation even if the patient is clinically improved.

- Prophylaxis. There are 2 types of prophylaxis for SBP—primary and secondary. In primary prophylaxis, patients at high risk for development of SBP should be given prophylactic antibiotics. There are 2 known high-risk groups—cirrhotic patients with acute GI bleeding and cirrhotic patients with very low protein ascites (< 1.0 g/dL).[1,5,17,19] **All patients with ascites and acute GI bleeding should be given antibiotics for 7 days (usually a fluoroquinolone) to help prevent the development of SBP.**[1,19] In secondary prophylaxis, patients with a history of SBP should remain on lifelong antibiotic prophylaxis to prevent another episode.[5,17,19] The likelihood of recurrent SBP is 70% without prophylaxis.[17] Different prophylactic strategies exist, including ciprofloxacin 750 mg PO weekly or ciprofloxacin 500 mg PO daily. We prefer daily dosing, as do multiple sources.[1,13,17,19]

WHAT TO DO IF THE TREATMENT ALGORITHM IS INEFFECTIVE

This section will be comprised of treatment modalities that are considered second line of emerging therapies.

Ascites Second-Line Treatments

Serial Paracentesis

Up to 17% of patients with ascites will develop refractory ascites.[13] This is defined as a patient who continues to have symptomatic ascites on maximal doses of diuretics, recurs rapidly after therapeutic paracentesis, or is intolerant to diuretics.[1,13,19] In this population, serial paracentesis is the next therapeutic option.[13] These are typically performed as an outpatient and can also be performed under ultrasound guidance.[14] If more than 5 L is to be removed, it is recommended that the patient receive IV albumin (8 g albumin/L of ascites removed) to help prevent postparacentesis circulatory dysfunction and development of HRS.[1,2,13] Preferably, the albumin should be infusing during the procedure.

Transjugular Intrahepatic Portosystemic Shunt

If a patient is requiring paracentesis more than weekly, consideration should be given to transjugular intrahepatic portosystemic shunts (TIPS).[1,5] TIPS is superior to serial paracentesis for the management of refractory ascites but does not offer survival benefit.[1,2,5,20] TIPS is a procedure performed by interventional radiologists during which a connection is created between a branch of the hepatic vein and a branch of the portal vein. The hepatic veins are accessed via the right internal jugular vein and a stent is placed over a wire, through the liver, connecting the pre- and posthepatic circulation.[21]

Transhepatic gradients are measured before and after placement of a TIPS, with the goal to decrease the gradient below 12 mm Hg.[21] To have a TIPS placed, the patient must have patent portal and hepatic veins and no known right heart failure or significant pulmonary hypertension. The TIPS will create a higher preload seen by the right atrium and could precipitate heart failure if predisposing factors exist.[19,21] Therefore, a duplex examination of the liver and a transthoracic echocardiogram should be performed before considering a TIPS. Another consideration before placing a TIPS is hepatic encephalopathy (HE). By bypassing the intrahepatic circulation, TIPS creates a predisposition for HE,[20] possibly by increasing ammonia concentration to the brain.[21] Thus, TIPS is not a good option for patients with preexisting HE or recurrent HE. Morbidity and mortality after TIPS have been correlated to model for end-stage liver disease (MELD) scores.[22,23] Patients with higher MELD scores have higher mortality post-TIPS, particularly MELD > 18. **Ideal TIPS candidates are those with refractory ascites and relatively preserved synthetic function, no concomitant heart failure, and patent perihepatic vasculature.**[5,24]

Other Peritoneovenous Shunts

Other surgical shunts have been performed historically for refractory ascites, including the LeVeen and Denver shunts. Though they are effective in managing ascites, these procedures have not been shown to improve mortality and are associated with increased surgical morbidity.[1,9] They are not commonly performed today.[13] They should be considered only by an experienced surgeon in a situation where a patient with refractory ascites cannot receive a transplant, TIPS, or serial paracentesis.[1]

Special Situation—Hyponatremia and Ascites

Dilutional hyponatremia occurs in approximately 20% of patients with cirrhosis as a result of ADH release leading to free water retention.[13] Hyponatremia is an independent predictor of poor outcome in cirrhosis and is associated with HRS type 2 and HE.[4,5,13] There are few effective treatments for hyponatremia in patients with cirrhosis, though it does not always require treatment. In fact, correction of the hyponatremia can sometimes create more complications than the hyponatremia itself.[1] **Diuretics are usually discontinued when serum sodium is < 130 mmol/L.**[13] **Fluid restriction is recommended in patients with sodium ≤ 125 mmol/L.**[1]

A new class of drugs called the *aquaretics* has shown promise in treating dilutional hyponatremia by activating aquaporin channels in the kidney to promote water excretion.[1,5] IV (conivaptan) and oral (tolvaptan) agents are now available in the United States. Both are currently only being used in hospitalized patients, with close electrolyte monitoring. Discontinuation of the fluid restriction while taking these medications is imperative to prevent central pontine myelinolysis from rapid sodium correction. Long-term safety of these new agents, effects of concurrent administration with diuretics, and cost-effectiveness are still unknown; however, this class of drugs is promising for future management of ascites and hyponatremia.[1,5]

HEPATORENAL SYNDROME SECOND-LINE TREATMENTS

Systemic Vasoconstrictors (Terlipressin, Vasopressin, Norepinephrine)

Terlipressin has been extensively studied in HRS but has yet to acquire Food and Drug Administration (FDA) approval in the United States.[4] It works by increasing vascular endothelial vasoconstriction (V1 receptor) and exhibits some effect on increasing water retention (V2 receptor).[16] It has a greater affinity for the V1 receptor than other available vasoconstrictive agents and is administered by IV in intermittent doses 0.5 to 1.0 mg every 4 to 6 h in combination with albumin infusions.[11] If the patient is tolerating terlipressin and the creatinine has not decreased within 2 days to 30% of the starting value, the dose should be increased.[4,16] It can be titrated up to 2 mg every 4 to 6 h until serum creatinine improves. Approximately 50% of patients treated with terlipressin have a good response, and the survival benefit is increased in those who respond to treatment.[25,26] However, 40% of patients do not respond to the treatment and it cannot be used in patient with preexisting cardiovascular disorders.[4] Additionally, HRS recurs in up to half of patients treated with terlipressin upon withdrawal.[4,11] A recent meta-analysis suggested that terlipressin, in combination with albumin, is effective in improving short-term (15-day) mortality in patients with HRS type 1 but does not promote longer term survival.[26] It may be an ideal drug to use in HRS type 1 as a bridge to transplant when safe to use and available. Little data are available on terlipressin in HRS type 2.

Vasopressin has been tried in patients with HRS in countries where terlipressin is not available.[16] Either alone or in combination with octreotide, 40% of patients in one retrospective study had improvement in renal function.[27] Vasopressin, a systemic and splanchnic vasoconstrictor, is given by continuous IV infusion and thus can usually only be used by inpatients in the intensive care unit in the United States. The use of vasopressin, a potent vasoconstrictor, involves the risk of inducing cardiac or intestinal ischemia. Thus, it must be used with great caution; many have used concurrent nitrates to mitigate such effects.

Norepinephrine has also been studied in small studies via continuous infusion of 0.5 to 3.0 mg/h, with concomitant episodic albumin infusions, with the goal to increase the mean arterial pressure by $\geq$ 10 mm Hg.[12] This therapy, too, requires administration in an inpatient intensive care setting in the United States. In small studies comparing norepinephrine plus albumin versus terlipressin and albumin, both therapies were similarly effective in reversing creatinine.[16] Withdrawal of norepinephrine also led to recurrent HRS nearly half the time.[4] Heightened awareness for cardiovascular events is necessary while on vasoconstrictor agents.

Other Pharmacologic Therapies

Dopamine has been studied and is not effective in reversal of HRS and demonstrates no survival benefit.[4,12,16] Other classes of drugs including endothelin-1 antagonists and natriuretic peptides are also ineffective.[16]

Nonpharmacologic Therapies (TIPS, Artificial Hepatic Support Devices)

TIPS is a tempting therapy because it allows for reversal of portal hypertension, the first physiologic abnormality in a cascade of events that eventually lead to HRS.[4] Unfortunately, most patients with HRS are not candidates for TIPS secondary to elevated MELD score, encephalopathy, or cardiac dysfunction.[4] Though considered experimental in HRS, in a select group of patients with Child's A or B cirrhosis, low MELD score, no known cardiac disease, and no encephalopathy, TIPS could be considered in patients with HRS who fail to respond to volume expansion and vasoconstrictor therapies.[13,24] This would likely be in the setting of a clinical trial, however.

- Artificial hepatic support devices. Many devices, including the Molecular Adsorbent Recirculating System (MARS) and albumin-based liver dialysis devices, have been developed for use in patients with decompensated cirrhosis.[11,16] These are typically available only at selected transplant centers. They have been shown to decrease creatinine values, but their clinical impact and utility are still unknown.[11,13,16] Further research is currently ongoing in this area.
- Renal replacement therapy (RRT). Dialysis is typically reserved for patients with HRS type 1 who are listed for liver transplantation or attempting evaluation for transplantation.[3] RRT does not improve the prognosis of HRS, but it can be helpful in managing the complications of HRS, including volume overload, acidosis, and electrolyte abnormalities.[1,4,5,8,12,16] With few exceptions, RRT is not justified in patients with terminal liver failure who are not transplant candidates.[16]

PREVENTION OF HEPATORENAL SYNDROME IN SPECIFIC SITUATIONS

Because no single treatment for HRS is completely effective, prevention of HRS is even more important. There are 3 situations in which a specific therapy has effectively decreased the incidence of HRS development in small trials (Table 5-4).[4]

Table 5-4

Specific Diagnoses Where Hepatorenal Syndrome Development May Be Prevented

Condition	Treatment
Alcoholic hepatitis	Pentoxifylline 400 mg PO tid
Spontaneous bacterial peritonitis	Albumin 1.5 g/kg IV on day 1 and 1 g/kg IV on day 3
Low protein ascites (ascitic protein < 1.5 g/dL)	Norfloxacin once daily (renally dosed)
PO indicates by mouth; tid, three times daily; IV, intravenous	

- Alcoholic hepatitis. Pentoxifylline 400 mg by mouth 3 times per day prevented HRS and improved in-hospital mortality in patients with severe alcoholic hepatitis (Maddrey discriminant function ≥ 32).[28]
- SBP. Infusion of albumin 1.5 g/kg IV on day 1 and 1 g/kg IV on day 3 in patients with SBP decreased the incidence of HRS and improved 3-month survival.[29]
- Low-protein ascites. In patients with ascitic protein concentration < 1.5 g/dL, daily prophylaxis with norfloxacin decreased the incidence of HRS and SBP and improved 3-month and 1-year survival.[30]

Additionally, avoidance of potentially nephrotoxic drugs, including iodinated contrast media, and prophylactic variceal treatment preventing variceal hemorrhage can help prevent HRS.

DISCUSSION ON WHEN TO REFER PATIENT TO A SPECIALTY GROUP

Any patient with ascites or HRS warrants referral to a transplant hepatologist, provided that he or she does not have any contraindications to liver transplantation (see Chapter 10).[31] **With few exceptions, the development of ascites should clue the provider in to the possibility that liver transplantation may be necessary, because there is an estimated 50% mortality at 2 years from its onset.**[2] These exceptions include the actively drinking patient with alcohol-related cirrhosis who could possibly reverse ascites by abstinence and the patient with acute hepatitis B who may recover with antiviral treatment.[1,9] Though ascites can often be managed effectively by the primary care physician, referral to a specialist before the development of refractory ascites may facilitate a well-paced transplant evaluation. Late referrals are often expedited and even done in the inpatient setting, contributing to increased cost of health care while exposing patients to possible nosocomial infections. Certainly, patients with refractory ascites are best managed in cooperation with a gastroenterologist or hepatologist.

HRS is most often managed in the hospital setting and should prompt a quick consultation by a liver specialist. As discussed above, no single therapy is completely effective for reversal of HRS other than liver transplantation. Therefore, HRS should not be managed solely by the primary care physician. Liver transplantation is the best option for patients with HRS type 1 or 2.[1,4,11,16] If performed early in the disease course, liver transplantation without kidney transplantation can usually be performed with similar outcomes to patients undergoing liver transplantation for reasons other than HRS.[4] If RRT has been initiated, or the disease has been present for more than 8 weeks, combined liver/kidney transplantation may be necessary.[4] Always consult with a nephrologist before deciding whether a patient needs single or dual organ transplantation, because some patients with HRS may have a concomitant intrinsic renal disease and dual organ transplantation may be preferred. Because creatinine is the highest weighted factor in the MELD scoring system, patients with HRS are often transplanted quickly after diagnosis.[11] All of the above therapies for HRS are utilized to prolong survival while awaiting transplantation.

REFERENCES

1. Runyon BA. AASLD practice guidelines: management of adult patients with ascites due to cirrhosis: an update. *Hepatology.* 2009;49:2087-2107.
2. Moore KP, Aithal GP. Guidelines on the management of ascites in cirrhosis. *Gut.* 2006;55 (suppl 6):vi1-vi12.
3. Gines P, Cardenas A, Arroyo V, Rodes J. Management of cirrhosis and ascites. *N Engl J Med.* 2004;350:1646-1654.
4. Munoz SJ. The hepatorenal syndrome. *Med Clin North Am.* 2008;92:viii-ix,813-837.
5. Sanyal AJ, Bosch J, Blei A, Arroyo V. Portal hypertension and its complications. *Gastroenterology.* 2008;134:1715-1728.
6. Angeli P, Merkel C. Pathogenesis and management of hepatorenal syndrome in patients with cirrhosis. *J Hepatol.* 2008;48(suppl 1):S93-S103.
7. Stadlbauer V, Wright GA, Banaji M, et al. Relationship between activation of the sympathetic nervous system and renal blood flow autoregulation in cirrhosis. *Gastroenterology.* 2008;134:111-119.
8. Mackelaite L, Alsauskas ZC, Ranganna K. Renal failure in patients with cirrhosis. *Med Clin N Am.* 2009;93:855-869.
9. Hou W, Sanyal AJ. Ascites: diagnosis and management. *Med Clin N Am.* 2009;93:801-817.
10. Noone TC, Semelka RC, Chaney DM, Reinhold C. Abdominal imaging studies: comparison of diagnostic accuracies resulting from ultrasound, computed tomography, and magnetic resonance imaging in the same individual. *Magn Reson Imaging.* 2004;22:19-24.
11. Salerno F, Gerbes A, Gines P, Wong F, Arroyo V. Diagnosis, prevention and treatment of hepatorenal syndrome in cirrhosis. *Gut.* 2007;56:1310-1318.
12. Gines P, Schrier RW. Renal failure in cirrhosis. *N Engl J Med.* 2009;361:1279-1290.
13. Garcia-Tsao G, Lim J. Management and treatment of patients with cirrhosis and portal hypertension: recommendations from the department of Veterans Affairs Hepatitis C resource center program and the National Hepatitis C program. *Am J Gastroenterol.* 2009;104:1802-1829.

14. Wong CL, Holroyd-Leduc J, Thorpe KE, Straus SE. Does this patient have bacterial peritonitis or portal hypertension? How do I perform a paracentesis and analyze the results? *JAMA*. 2008;299:1166-1178.

15. Mimidis K, Papadopoulos V, Kartalis G. Eplerenone relieves spironolactone-induced painful gynaecomastia in patients with decompensated hepatitis B–related cirrhosis. *Scand J Gastroenterol*. 2007;42:1516-1517.

16. Kiser TH, MacLaren R, Fish DN. Treatment of hepatorenal syndrome. *Pharmacotherapy*. 2009;29:1196-1211.

17. Koulaouzidis A, Bhat S, Saeed AA. Spontaneous bacterial peritonitis. *World J Gastroenterol*. 2009;15:1042-1049.

18. Kim YS, Kestell MF, Lee SP. Gall-bladder sludge: lessons from ceftriaxone. *J Gastroenterol Hepatol*. 1992;7:618-621.

19. Lee JM, Han KH, Ahn SH. Ascites and spontaneous bacterial peritonitis: an Asian perspective. *J Gastroenterol Hepatol*. 2009;24:1494-1503.

20. Saab S, Nieto JM, Lewis SK, Runyon BA. TIPS versus paracentesis for cirrhotic patients with refractory ascites. *Cochrane Database Syst Rev*. 2006;4:CD004889.

21. Owen AR, Stanley AJ, Vijayananthan A, Moss JG. The transjugular intrahepatic portosystemic shunt (TIPS). *Clin Radiol*. 2009;64:664-667.

22. Schepke M, Roth F, Fimmers R, et al. Comparison of MELD, Child-Pugh, and Emory model for the prediction of survival in patients undergoing transjugular intrahepatic portosystemic shunting. *Am J Gastroenterol*. 2003;98:1167-1174.

23. Ferral H, Gamboa P, Postoak DW, et al. Survival after elective transjugular intrahepatic portosystemic shunt creation: prediction with model for end-stage liver disease score. *Radiology*. 2004;231:231-236.

24. Senzolo M, Cholongitas E, Tibballs J, Burroughs A, Patch D. Transjugular intrahepatic portosystemic shunt in the management of ascites and hepatorenal syndrome. *Eur J Gastroenterol Hepatol*. 2006;18:1143-1150.

25. Fabrizi F, Dixit V, Martin P. Meta-analysis: terlipressin therapy for the hepatorenal syndrome. *Aliment Pharmacol Ther*. 2006;24:935-944.

26. Sanyal AJ, Boyer T, Garcia-Tsao G, et al. A randomized, prospective, double-blind, placebo-controlled trial of terlipressin for type 1 hepatorenal syndrome. *Gastroenterology*. 2008;134:1360-1368.

27. Kiser TH, Fish DN, Obritsch MD, Jung R, MacLaren R, Parikh CR. Vasopressin, not octreotide, may be beneficial in the treatment of hepatorenal syndrome: a retrospective study. *Nephrol Dial Transpl*. 2005;20:1813-1820.

28. Akriviadis E, Botla R, Briggs W, Han S, Reynolds T, Shakil O. Pentoxifylline improves short-term survival in severe acute alcoholic hepatitis: a double-blind, placebo-controlled trial. *Gastroenterology*. 2000;119:1637-1648.

29. Sort P, Navasa M, Arroyo V, et al. Effect of intravenous albumin on renal impairment and mortality in patients with cirrhosis and spontaneous bacterial peritonitis. *N Engl J Med*. 1999;341:403-409.

30. Fernández J, Navasa M, Planas R, et al. Primary prophylaxis of spontaneous bacterial peritonitis delays hepatorenal syndrome and improves survival in cirrhosis. *Gastroenterology*. 2007;133:818-824.

31. O'Leary JG, Lepe R, Davis GL. Indications for liver transplantation. *Gastroenterology*. 2008;134:1765-1776.

chapter 6

MANAGEMENT OF
HEPATIC ENCEPHALOPATHY

Jayant A. Talwalkar, MD, MPH

Hepatic encephalopathy (HE) may be defined as a disturbance in central nervous system function because of hepatic insufficiency. This broad definition reflects the existence of a spectrum of neuropsychiatric manifestations related to a range of pathophysiologic mechanisms. Present in both acute and chronic liver failure, these neuropsychiatric manifestations are potentially reversible.[1,2]

EPIDEMIOLOGY, CLASSIFICATION, AND CLINICAL MANIFESTATIONS

Epidemiology

Approximately 5.5 million persons in the United States have cirrhosis of the liver, a major cause of complications and death. Overt episodes of HE are debilitating, can occur without warning, render the patient incapable of self-care, and frequently result in hospitalization.[3] In 2004, an estimated 50,000 patients were hospitalized with HE.[4] Although the occurrence of episodes of HE appears to be unrelated to the cause of cirrhosis, increases in the frequency and severity of such episodes predict an increased risk of death.[5]

Classification

The classification of HE has been centered around terminology that has been proposed to identify the clinical manifestations of this syndrome.[6]

Zaman A. *Managing the Complications of Cirrhosis: A Practical Approach* (pp 77-88).
© 2012 Taylor & Francis Group.

Table 6-1

West Haven Criteria for the Diagnosis of Hepatic Encephalopathy

Stage	Distinguishing Features
0	No abnormality detected
1	Trivial lack of awareness
	Euphoria or anxiety
	Shortened attention span
	Impairment of addition or subtraction
2	Lethargy or apathy
	Disorientation for time
	Obvious personality change
	Inappropriate behavior
3	Somnolence to semi-stupor
	Responsive to stimuli
	Confused
	Gross disorientation
	Bizarre behavior
4	Coma, unable to test mental state

Development of an acute confusional state that can evolve into coma (acute encephalopathy) is the most overt manifestation of HE. Patients with fulminant hepatic failure as well as cirrhosis can present with signs and symptoms associated with acute encephalopathy. In patients with cirrhosis, acute encephalopathy is most commonly associated with a precipitating factor that triggers the change in mental state.[1,2] Recurrent episodes can occur without a precipitating factor, or the neurologic deficits may not completely reverse even with therapy. The most frequent neurologic disturbances are mild cognitive abnormalities defined recently as minimal hepatic encephalopathy (MHE) and are only found with structured psychometric testing.[1,7]

Clinical Manifestations

The West Haven criteria were developed years ago to categorize the clinical manifestations of HE, as well as to provide a way for assessing the severity of involvement in affected patients (Table 6-1). Stage 0 HE can apply to individuals with normal cognitive function as well as those with minimal HE.[1,7] Furthermore, the ability to discriminate between stage 0 and stage 1 may be

---

Table 6-2

Diagnostic Tests for Hepatic Encephalopathy

Serum ammonia level
Psychometric testing (PHES, CFF)
Neurophysiological testing (EEG)
Computed tomography (for porto-systemic shunts)
Magnetic resonance imaging (also MR spectroscopy)
PHES indicates psychometric hepatic encephalopathy test score; CFF, critical flicker frequency; EEG, electroencephalography; MRI, magnetic resonance

difficult because criteria for both categories may be found together in the same patient. Patients with stage 2 HE are generally confused and often require urgent medical evaluation and subsequent hospitalization for treatment.

MHE is defined as cognitive dysfunction without clinical signs of overt HE.[6-8] The main reason to investigate the presence of MHE is to advise patients with cirrhosis who are at risk for accidents, such as active drivers, those with a decline in work performance, or those who complain of cognitive symptoms. There is no evidence of long-term memory or language function decline in patients with MHE. The diagnosis of MHE usually requires specialized psychometric testing, yet this is often impractical within the confines of ambulatory clinical practice unless a trained neuropsychologist is available. However, this evaluation is not easy to carry out due to its costs, complexity, and length. Therefore, until simple and practical diagnostic tools for MHE are available for the practicing clinician, this entity is still is in its infancy and will not be covered further in this book.

DIAGNOSIS

Table 6-2 lists some typical diagnostic tests for HE. However, the diagnosis of HE first requires excluding other potential causes for encephalopathy.[1] Metabolic disorders, infectious diseases, intracranial vascular events, and intracranial space-occupying lesions can present with similar neuropsychiatric symptomatology and need to be excluded.[1]

Possible alterations of the hepatic circulation may also be contributing factors for the development of HE. In a recent study, Riggio and colleagues[9] assessed the incidence, natural history, and risk factors of HE after transjugular intrahepatic porto-systemic shunt (TIPS). Among 78 patients treated by TIPS with polytetrafluoroethylene (PTFE)-covered stent grafts, at least one episode of HE occurred in 45% within a 2-year period. Over 50% of cases were defined as severe HE (stage 3 or 4 by West Haven criteria). The development of refractory HE in 6 patients required shunt diameter reduction to improve symptoms. Risk factors were older age, high creatinine levels, low serum sodium, and low albumin values. The association between HE and large spontaneous porto-systemic shunts has also been reported.[10] Cirrhotic patients with persistent or recurrent HE commonly have large spontaneous portal-systemic shunts. Using multidetector computed tomography (CT) imaging, large spontaneous porto-systemic shunts were significantly more common in patients with (71%) than without (14%) HE.[10] This approach is most ideal in patients with compensated liver disease where signs and symptoms suggest HE but the severity of liver disease is mild.

The measurement of serum ammonia levels for the diagnosis of HE remains controversial. No significant correlation between serum ammonia level and stage of HE has been observed. Most authorities would agree that measurement of ammonia may be helpful in the initial evaluation of unexplained encephalopathy in patients with no known prior history of liver disease. Normal ammonia values in these patients would argue against a diagnosis of HE. If ammonia levels are to be measured, the use of arterial blood is preferred. Follow-up with repeated ammonia levels is unnecessary and does not replace the evaluation of the patient's mental state.[1]

Electroencephalography (EEG) is often performed in patients with their first presentation of HE or in any patient in whom the presentation is atypical in nature. The EEG may have some value in determining the advanced stages of HE when characteristic triphasic waves are identified. However, the correlation between EEG with psychometric measures like the psychometric hepatic encephalopathy test score (PHES) is poor.[7] There is no clear role for evoked potential measurement in the clinical setting.

Magnetic resonance imaging of the brain has become a standard technique for the assessment of patients with neurologic manifestations.[2] Patients with cirrhosis and no clinical manifestations of HE can have symmetrical high-signal abnormalities in the pallidum on T1-weighted images.[11,12] Pallidal hyperintensity is not related to the grade of HE; rather, its absence in a patient with cirrhosis and neurologic manifestations suggests an alternative diagnosis.[8] An accumulation of manganese may explain the T1 abnormality.[12] Decreased brain myo-inositol and elevated glutamine by magnetic resonance spectroscopy is characteristic of HE when detected. Neither cutoff values nor the diagnostic accuracy of this pattern has been established, however.[12] Currently, there is no established clinical role for positron emission tomography (PET) scanning in the diagnosis of HE.

TREATMENT

Several treatment goals have been described for the management of HE, which includes the following categories[1]:

Provision of Supportive Care

Mental status changes can be rapid, with disorientation potentially causing harm to patients and caregivers. The prevention of falls with early HE requires special measures, including assistance for patients when they are ambulating. In deeper stages of HE, the need for prophylactic tracheal intubations needs to be considered.[1]

Identification of Precipitating Factors

In most cases of cirrhosis with acute or chronic HE, a precipitating factor is found during investigations. **Major categories of precipitants include (1) gastrointestinal hemorrhage; (2) infection with specific reference to spontaneous bacterial peritonitis or pneumonia; (3) electrolyte disturbances including metabolic alkalosis, hypokalemia, dehydration, and diuretic effects; (4) the use of psychoactive medications including benzodiazepines, narcotics, and other sedatives; (5) constipation; (6) excessive dietary protein (in rare cases); and (7) acute deterioration of liver function in cirrhosis from superimposed alcoholic hepatitis, the development of an acute circulatory disturbance (eg, portal vein thrombosis), recent surgery, or TIPS placement. Spontaneous encephalopathy (no precipitant factor identified) should raise the suspicion of an abnormal collateral circulation.[1,2]**

Reduction of Excess Nitrogen in the Gut

Bowel cleansing reduces the luminal content of ammonia, decreases colonic bacterial counts, and lowers blood ammonia in cirrhotic patients.[1] Various laxatives may be used, but nonabsorbable disaccharides or antibiotics may be more effective because they result in additional effects that potentiate the elimination or reduce the formation of nitrogenous compounds (see below). Administration of nonabsorbable disaccharide enemas may be necessary in the patient with hepatic coma.

Lactulose

Lactulose is a nonabsorbable disaccharide that decreases the absorption of ammonia through cathartic effects and subsequent acidification of the colon (ie, lower pH). Passage of ammonia into the colonic lumen results in its incorporation into bacteria with a resulting decrease of portal blood ammonia. As a result, peripheral levels of ammonia are reduced and the total body pool of urea decreases.

For acute encephalopathy, lactulose (ingested or via nasogastric tube), 45 mL orally, is followed by dosing every hour until bowel evacuation occurs. Dosing frequency is then reduced to obtain 2 to 3 soft bowel movements per day (generally 15 to 45 mL every 8 to 12 h). Lactulose by enema (300 mL in 1 L of water) is retained for 1 h, with the patient in the Trendelenburg position (to increase the possibility of access to the right colon).[1]

For chronic encephalopathy, oral dosing of lactulose can begin with 15 to 30 cc orally 1 to 2 times daily. Increased dosing through more frequent ingestion (ie, every 6 to 8 h) may be required to achieve 2 to 3 soft formed bowel movements every 24 h.[1]

Lactulose has been associated with a number of adverse effects, including nausea, vomiting, abdominal cramping, and unpalatability due to its excessively sweet taste. Mixing lactulose with small amounts of juice or water may help to improve its palatability. Greater than 3 bowel movements per day and/or watery diarrhea require a reduction in dosing. Patients should not be encouraged to stop using lactulose altogether when side effects develop but to taper lactulose use to its lowest effective dose if possible. Lactulose can be used in patients with lactase deficiency.[12]

The efficacy of lactulose, and subsequently its position as a standard of care, has recently been questioned. A recent meta-analysis investigated the effect of nonabsorbable disaccharides (lactulose or lacitol) compared with placebo, antibiotics, or no intervention.[13] The main result was that nonabsorbable disaccharides are inferior to antibiotics for the treatment of HE. The analysis of the 2 high-quality trials (44 patients) that compared nonabsorbable disaccharides to placebo found no significant effect, whereas lesser quality trials found a beneficial effect for lactulose. Despite these observations, the data on the biological effects of these compounds and a large clinical experience remain sufficient to justify their use.[1,2] For example, a recent study identified better cognitive function and health-related quality of life in patients with cirrhosis and MHE.[14]

Nonabsorbable Oral Antibiotics

Antibiotics are a therapeutic alternative to nonabsorbable disaccharides for treatment in acute and chronic HE in patients with cirrhosis. The most common antibiotics used for HE are neomycin, metronidazole, and, more recently, rifaxamin.

The mechanism of action for neomycin in HE is associated with reducing the effects of colonic bacteria on ammonia production. However, neomycin will also affect the small bowel mucosa and may impair the activity of glutaminase in intestinal villi. Metronidazole, which affects a different bacterial population than neomycin within the colonic flora, will also improve HE by reducing ammonia production. Recently, infection with *Helicobacter pylori* was proposed as a mechanism responsible for encephalopathy, in view of the generation of ammonia by this urease-containing organism. A careful assessment of its eradication failed to show a distinct impact on mental states or blood ammonia levels in patients with MHE. Thus, the eradication of *H. pylori* cannot be recommended as a therapeutic strategy.[1,2]

Both neomycin and metronidazole have associated side effects when used long term. Despite its poor absorption, chronic neomycin may cause auditory loss and renal failure. It has been suggested that patients require annual auditory testing if maintained on chronic neomycin. Intestinal malabsorption can result in a spruelike diarrhea. Metronidazole neurotoxicity can be severe in patients with cirrhosis, where impaired clearance of the drug may be present. Symptoms may include peripheral neuropathy and a metallic-like taste.[1,2]

For the treatment of acute HE, neomycin (3 to 6 g/day orally) can be given for a period of 1 to 2 weeks. For chronic HE, neomycin (1 to 2 g/day orally) should be given, with periodic renal and annual auditory monitoring. Metronidazole should be started at a dose of 250 mg orally twice a day. Both neomycin and metronidazole can be combined with oral lactulose in problematic cases of patients who are intolerant of higher doses of lactulose.

Rifaximin

Rifaximin is a minimally absorbed oral antibiotic with activity against gram-positive and gram-negative aerobic and anaerobic enteric bacteria. In randomized studies mainly from Europe and Asia, rifaximin has been found to be more effective than lactulose or lacitol. Furthermore, rifaximin was observed to have equivalent or greater efficacy when compared to other antibiotics in patients with acute HE.[15]

Recently, a large randomized, double-blind, placebo-controlled trial was conducted among 299 patients in remission from recurrent HE (defined as ≥ 2 episodes within the previous 6 months) in association with chronic liver disease. Patients were randomized to receive either rifaximin 550 mg orally twice a day (140 patients) or placebo (159 patients) for 6 months. The primary study end point was measured by the time to the first breakthrough episode of HE, and a major secondary end point was the time to first hospitalization involving HE. Notably, the use of rifaximin significantly reduced the risk of an episode of HE compared to placebo by 58% over a 6-month period. A breakthrough episode of HE occurred in 22% of patients in the rifaximin group, compared to 46% of patients in the placebo group. Fourteen percent of rifaximin-treated patients were hospitalized for HE during the study, compared to 23% of patients in the placebo group. More than 90% of patients received concomitant lactulose therapy, with similar average daily doses observed between rifaximin and placebo-treated groups. The current study differs from previous randomized studies in that it examined the protective effect of rifaximin against breakthrough episodes of HE rather than its effect in the treatment of acute, overt symptoms; the study also involved a larger group of patients and a longer study period.[15] As a result of this large randomized trial, rifaximin 550 mg orally twice a day was given regulatory approval for use in patients with HE by the US Food and Drug Administration (FDA). **A reasonable clinical approach would be to initially start with lactulose titrated to 2 to 3 bowel movements a day. If this inadequately controls HE (recurrent HE episodes or hospitalizations for HE), adding rifaximin 550 mg twice daily should be the next step. Furthermore, if the patient becomes intolerant or noncompliant with lactulose, switching to rifaximin should be the next step. Alternatives, such as neomycin and metronidazole, should be avoided due to their long-term side effects and toxicities.**

Providing Adequate Nutritional Support

Traditionally, protein restriction was strongly advocated for patients with HE. However, the basis for protein restriction has been anecdotal. Furthermore, protein restriction may be associated with an increased mortality risk when compared to patients without protein-restricted diets. In patients with episodic HE, the only randomized trial that has been conducted did not find differences in the outcome of HE between a low-protein and a normal protein diet. Protein restriction favors protein degradation, and if maintained for long periods worsens the nutritional status. Though a high content of proteins in the diet induces hyperammonemia and may precipitate HE, this is a relatively uncommon event. **Thus, protein restriction is no longer recommended.**[1,2]

Zinc, which is a cofactor of urea cycle enzymes, may be deficient in patients with cirrhosis and especially among individuals with significant muscle wasting and malnutrition. Zinc supplementation improves the activity of the urea cycle in experimental models of cirrhosis, and additional human studies suggest that it may have incremental beneficial effects in temporizing the symptoms associated with HE.[1,2]

In the treatment of acute HE, it has been recommended that withdrawal of protein from the diet over the first 1 to 2 days is reasonable. Short-term (< 5 days) enteral nutrition has not been shown to benefit hospitalized cirrhotic patients. Once patients have recovered from the acute HE episode, they can resume an oral diet (if cognition is satisfactory) that contains protein. In patients with chronic HE, the amount of daily protein recommended is 1 to 1.5 g protein/kg/day. Vegetable and dairy sources may be preferable to animal protein, because they provide a higher calorie-to-nitrogen ratio and, in the case of vegetable protein, provide nonabsorbable fiber, which may help to increase subsequent colonic acidification. Furthermore, vegetable and dairy protein may be preferred because some patients with cirrhosis have described losing their taste for meats like beef and chicken. Oral formulation of branched-chain amino acids may provide a better tolerated source of protein in patients with chronic HE and dietary protein intolerance. Zinc acetate or zinc sulfate can be administered at initial doses of 220 mg orally twice a day. If tolerated, this can be given up to 4 times a day, yet gastrointestinal side effects like nausea may limit the ability to reach this dosing frequency.[1,2]

Assessment of the Need for Long-Term Therapy

Patients with cirrhosis are at risk of developing recurrent episodes of HE. **Therefore, the ability to prevent recurrence of potential precipitating factors is crucial. These include the avoidance of dehydration, avoidance of constipation, prophylaxis of bleeding from gastroesophageal varices, prophylaxis of spontaneous bacterial peritonitis, the judicious use of diuretics, and avoidance of psychoactive medications.**[1] When patients develop HE in the absence of a precipitating factor, health care providers are also required to determine whether noncompliance or the inability to tolerate medications for HE has occurred. Prevention of a first episode of HE in subjects who have undergone a TIPS procedure is done in some centers by preemptively using lactulose, yet no controlled data are available to determine the efficacy of this strategy.

MANAGEMENT OF
REFRACTORY HEPATIC ENCEPHALOPATHY

Flumazenil

Flumazenil, a short-acting benzodiazepine receptor antagonist, has been used as a treatment for patients with HE. An enhanced gamma-aminobutyric acid (GABA)-ergic tone was postulated to contribute to the development of encephalopathy. It has been proposed that endogenous benzodiazepines may be present in patients with HE and exert neuroinhibitory effects via binding to the GABA$_A$ receptor. Antagonism of their effect with flumazenil has been tested in patients with acute encephalopathy and severe changes in mental state. There is evidence of an increase in benzodiazepine receptor activation among cirrhotic patients with HE. In a systematic review, Als-Nielsen and colleagues included 12 controlled trials with a total of 765 patients and found flumazenil to be associated with a significant improvement in HE.[13] It failed to show any long-term benefits or improvement in survival, however. Enthusiasm for using flumazenil is also hampered by side effects, including oversedation as well as agitation.[1,16]

Probiotic Therapy

Probiotic therapy modifies intestinal flora, decreases plasma ammonia, may diminish bacterial translocation, and might reduce the induction of inflammatory mediators. Probiotics have been used to treat HE by decreasing urease-producing bacteria and promoting the growth of non-urease-producing bacteria. Small clinical experiences have described reducing ammonia levels and improving cognitive function with probiotics in patients with minimal and chronic HE.

Manipulation of the Splanchnic Circulation

Large splenorenal or gastrorenal shunts may be amenable to occlusion via radiologic techniques, including placement of occlusive coils. Access to the portal circulation is best obtained through the transhepatic route. In this limited experience, no increased risk of variceal hemorrhage was observed after occlusion of the shunt. Occlusion of portal-systemic collaterals should be undertaken only in centers with experienced interventional radiologists and after all other medical measures have failed.[1,2,16]

Artificial Liver Support Devices

Liver support devices, such as the Molecular Adsorbent Recirculating System (MARS), might also play a role in the treatment of refractory HE. MARS is a blood detoxification system based on albumin dialysis. The system removes both protein-bound and water-soluble toxins, which makes it useful for patients with liver failure. The FDA has approved MARS as a toxin removal device in cases of drug overdose and poisoning; however, it is not yet approved for HE.[1,16] MARS improves the grade of HE independent of changes in ammonia and cytokines, suggesting that other toxins, such as oxygen-based free radicals, might be important.[2] A prospective, controlled, randomized multicenter trial in patients with HE (grade 3 or 4) was randomized to standard medical therapy or MARS dialysis with standard medical therapy. The MARS dialysis-treated group had a more significant and rapid improvement in their mental status compared to standard medical therapy.[16]

Liver Transplantation

The development of HE in patients with cirrhosis is associated with a survival lower than 50% at 2 years. For this reason, liver transplantation should be considered in these patients. Though the model for end-stage liver disease (MELD) system has been used to prioritize the allocation of organs, it may underestimate the prognosis of patients who develop HE. However, the MELD score may accurately reflect the expected survival in patients with recurrent

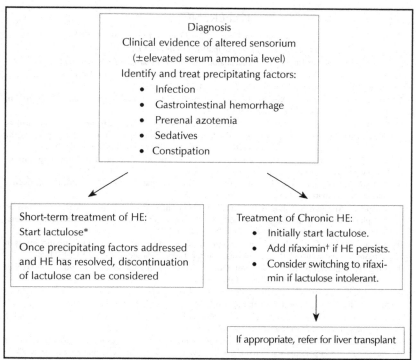

Figure 6-1. Practical approach to the diagnosis and treatment of hepatic encephalopathy (HE). *Lactulose dose titrated to 2 to 3 soft formed stools daily. †Rifaximin 550 mg twice daily.

HE associated with large spontaneous portal-systemic shunts and relatively preserved liver function.[2] Liver transplantation improves HE, even in patients with severe manifestations. Prospective studies that have assessed neuropsychologic function following liver transplantation have challenged the notion of complete reversibility of HE.[16,17]

INDICATIONS FOR SPECIALTY REFERRAL

The development of overt HE carries a poor prognosis, and it is recommended that patients be referred to liver transplant centers after the first episode of overt HE for evaluation. In addition, patients with recurrent episodes of HE despite initial treatment approaches to prevent recurrent HE may benefit from specialty consultation with a hepatologist. See Figure 6-1 for diagnostic and treatment algorithm.

88 *Chapter 6*

REFERENCES

1. Blei AT, Cordoba J. Hepatic encephalopathy. *Am J Gastroenterol.* 2001;96:1968-1976.
2. Córdoba J, Mínguez B. Hepatic encephalopathy. *Semin Liver Dis.* 2008;28:70-80.
3. Poordad FF. The burden of hepatic encephalopathy. *Aliment Pharmacol Ther.* 2007;25(suppl 1):3-9.
4. Leevy CB, Phillips JA. Hospitalizations during the use of rifaximin versus lactulose for the treatment of hepatic encephalopathy. *Dig Dis Sci.* 2007;52:737-741.
5. Bustamante J, Rimola A, Ventura PJ, et al. Prognostic significance of hepatic encephalopathy in patients with cirrhosis. *J Hepatol.* 1999;30:890-895.
6. Ferenci P, Lockwood A, Mullen K, Tarter R, Weissenborn K, Blei AT. Hepatic encephalopathy—definition, nomenclature, diagnosis, and quantification: final report of the working party at the 11th World Congresses of Gastroenterology, Vienna, 1998. *Hepatology.* 2002;35:716-721.
7. Bajaj JS, Wade JB, Sanyal AJ. Spectrum of neurocognitive impairment in cirrhosis: implications for the assessment of hepatic encephalopathy. *Hepatology.* 2009;50:2014-2021.
8. Ortiz M, Jacas C, Cordoba J. Minimal hepatic encephalopathy: diagnosis, clinical significance and recommendations. *J Hepatol.* 2005;42(suppl):S45-S53.
9. Riggio O, Angeloni S, Salvatori FM, et al. Incidence, natural history, and risk factors of hepatic encephalopathy after transjugular intrahepatic portosystemic shunt with polytetrafluoroethylene-covered stent grafts. *Am J Gastroenterol.* 2008;103:2738-2746.
10. Riggio O, Efrati C, Catalano C, et al. High prevalence of spontaneous portal-systemic shunts in persistent hepatic encephalopathy: a case-control study. *Hepatology.* 2005;42:1158-1165.
11. Ong JP, Aggarwal A, Krieger D, et al. Correlation between ammonia levels and the severity of hepatic encephalopathy. *Am J Med.* 2003;114:188-193.
12. Zeneroli ML, Cioni G, Vezzeli C, Ventura E. Globus pallidus alterations and brain atrophy in liver cirrhosis patients with encephalopathy. *Magn Res Imaging.* 1991;9:295-302.
13. Als-Nielsen B, Gluud LL, Gluud C. Non-absorbable disaccharides for hepatic encephalopathy: systematic review of randomised trials. *BMJ.* 2004;328:1046.
14. Prasad S, Dhiman RK, Duseja A, et al. Lactulose improves cognitive functions and health-related quality of life in patients with cirrhosis who have minimal hepatic encephalopathy. *Hepatology.* 2007;45:549-559.
15. Bass NM, Mullen KD, Sanyal A, et al. Rifaximin treatment in hepatic encephalopathy. *N Engl J Med.* 2010;362:1071-1081.
16. Al Sibae MR, McGuire BM. Current trends in the treatment of hepatic encephalopathy. *Ther Clin Risk Manag.* 2009;5:617-626.
17. Sotil EU, Gottstein J, Ayala E, Randolph C, Blei AT. Impact of preoperative overt hepatic encephalopathy on neurocognitive function after liver transplantation. *Liver Transpl.* 2009;15:184-192.

chapter

7

Management of Hepatocellular Carcinoma

Jonathan M. Schwartz, MD

Hepatocellular carcinoma (HCC) is the fifth most common malignancy in men and the eighth most common in women worldwide.[1] The disease has a high case fatality rate, resulting in an estimated 500,000 deaths annually worldwide, and is the third most common cause of cancer-related death.[2]

The incidence of HCC in the United States has increased over the past 3 decades.[3] HCC occurs in patients with chronic liver disease, most often in the setting of cirrhosis, and is now the leading cause of death among patients with compensated cirrhosis. Unlike most malignancies where prognosis is contingent upon tumor characteristics, the degree of hepatic reserve needs to be taken into consideration when assessing prognosis and the appropriate treatment approach in HCC.

Although survival in HCC is improved with early detection through screening and surveillance,[4,5] surveillance programs are variably implemented, and HCC is often diagnosed at a late stage.[6] Consequently, curative therapies such as liver transplantation and hepatic resection or ablation can only be applied in a minority of patients at the time of diagnosis.[6] Widespread incorporation of screening and surveillance practices will hopefully change the proportion of patients who are eligible for curative therapies.

This chapter will review the staging of HCC, treatment strategies, including surgery and locoregional and systemic therapies, as well as the systems used to assess response to chosen therapy.

Zaman A. *Managing the Complications of Cirrhosis: A Practical Approach* (pp 89-96).

STAGING OF HEPATOCELLULAR CARCINOMA

Important factors predicting survival in patients with HCC include patient performance status (as assessed by the Eastern Cooperative Oncology Group [ECOG] classification), tumor characteristics (size, number, invasion of the portal venous system, extrahepatic disease, alpha-fetoprotein [AFP]), and the severity of underlying liver disease (as assessed by the Child-Turcotte-Pugh [CTP] classification or the model of end-stage liver disease [MELD] score).

Several staging systems have been derived using multivariate analyses of potential risk factors over the past several decades in various geographic regions. The Barcelona Clinic Liver Cancer (BCLC) staging system is the only staging system that incorporates performance status and treatment allocation into the prognostic model.[7]

The Okuda system[8] was the first system to incorporate hepatic function using the CTP score, tumor burden, and serum AFP. A second staging system was derived by the Cancer of the Liver Italian Program (CLIP).[9] This staging system assigned points according to the number and location of tumor nodules as well as the degree of AFP elevation (greater or less than 400 ng/mL). Prospective validation of this system suggested that it was superior to the Okuda system for predicting survival. In a prospective analysis, the median survival rates for patients with CLIP stages 0, 1, 2, 3, 4, and 5 to 6 were 31, 27, 13, 8, 2, and 2 months, respectively.

The BCLC group has developed a validated prognostic system that incorporates patient performance status, severity of liver disease, and tumor parameters[7,10] (Figure 7-1). Determination of prognosis using the MELD scoring system in HCC patients has also been used as an accurate staging system in Asian patients, mostly with hepatitis B infection.[11] A comparison of prognostic systems among patients referred to a US tertiary medical center validated the performance characteristics of the BCLC staging system,[12] which is the staging system endorsed by this author.

Molecular gene expression profiles of HCC have been shown to be important determinates of survival,[13] and the use of expression profiles will likely aid in assessing prognosis and response to various therapies.

TREATMENT OF HEPATOCELLULAR CARCINOMA

Given the complexity of treatment options in patients with varying degrees of hepatic reserve, it is helpful for patients with HCC to be managed at centers with dedicated multidisciplinary teams that include hepatologists, transplant surgeons, surgical oncologists, interventional radiologists, body imaging radiologists, and oncologists. The choice of treatment modalities should take into consideration both tumor characteristics and liver function. Surgical options

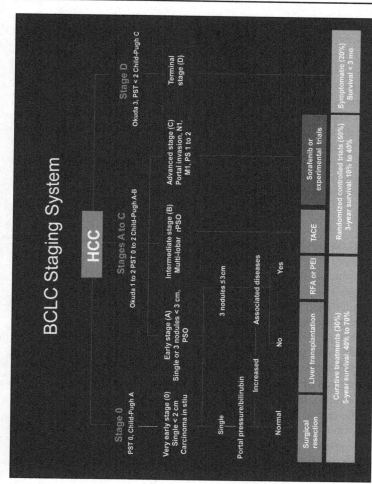

Figure 7-1. Barcelona Clinic Liver Cancer staging and treatment algorithm for hepatocellular carcinoma. (Adapted from Bruix J, Llovet JM. Major achievements in hepatocellular carcinoma. *Lancet.* 2009;373:614–616.)

(resection and liver transplantation) are favored and, when available, liver transplantation likely results in a highest probability of long-term survival. Other curative strategies include radiofrequency ablation (RFA) and percutaneous ethanol injection (PEI). Transarterial chemoembolization has also been demonstrated to improve survival in patients with more advanced HCC. Several other therapeutic methods, such as intra-arterial radiation and external beam radiation, are frequently used to treat HCC; however, these modalities have been subjected to less rigorous validation. The multikinase inhibitor sorafenib has recently been approved by regulatory agencies in the United States and Europe for treatment of advanced HCC. The BCLC treatment algorithm is a current representation of appropriate treatment strategies and survival rates based on implementation of these treatment approaches (see Figure 7-1).

LIVER RESECTION

In select patients with HCC, surgical resection can result in 5-year survival rates as high as 70%. Resection is typically tolerated in noncirrhotic patients with HCC, whereas patients with cirrhosis need to be carefully selected in order to reduce the risk of postoperative hepatic decompensation and subsequent morbidity and mortality.

Cirrhotic patients are candidates for surgical resection if they have preserved liver function (normal bilirubin) without portal hypertension (wedged hepatic portal venous pressure gradient of < 10 mm Hg) and a solitary HCC confined to the liver without radiographic evidence of hepatic vascular invasion.[14] There may be a benefit to surgical resection in patients with mild portal hypertension and vascular invasion of the tumor; however, the survival benefit is less pronounced.[15]

Although there is no specific size limitation for hepatic resection, large tumors are frequently associated with microvascular invasion and multifocal disease, which are risk factors for tumor recurrence. Improved preoperative imaging techniques and modalities such as intraoperative ultrasound to identify multifocal disease are helpful to improve patient selection.

The 5-year recurrence rate following resection of patients with HCC ranges from 38% to 68%, and the 5-year survival is approximately 30%. Five-year survival rates as high as 50% to 90% have been reported in carefully selected patients.[14,16] However, patients with underlying cirrhosis or chronic viral hepatitis remain at risk for recurrent disease and thus may have a less favorable prognosis.

Gene expression profiles of the nonmalignant surrounding hepatic parenchyma have been demonstrated to play an important role in determining the risk of long-term HCC recurrence.[17,18]

POSTOPERATIVE ADJUVANT THERAPIES

Postoperative chemotherapy or interferon does not provide a survival benefit. A trial using intrarterial iodinated lipiodol (131I-lipiodol) in Asian patients (mostly with hepatitis B infection) demonstrated lower rates of tumor recurrence and improved postoperative survival.[19] In addition, a Japanese trial using acyclic retinoids following hepatic resection reduced tumor recurrence and improved survival.[20] Limited availability has prevented widespread use of this agent. Targeted molecular therapies will possibly have a role in prevention of tumor recurrence following hepatic resection.

LIVER TRANSPLANTATION

Liver transplantation has the advantage of removing the tumor(s) and treating cirrhosis, which is considered a premalignant condition. Careful patient selection has improved recurrence-free survival. **Survival following liver transplantation for patients with tumors that meet the following criteria can exceed 70% at 5 years[21,22]:**

- **Solitary tumor 5 cm or less in diameter.**

- **No more than 3 tumor nodules, each less than 3 cm.**

- **No preoperative evidence of tumor invasion of blood vessels, lymph nodes, or extrahepatic metastasis.**

Achievement of such promising results depends on a short waiting period between the diagnosis of HCC and transplantation. Longer waiting periods can lead to tumor progression, with waiting list dropout rates as high as 25%.[23] In the United States, the United Network of Organ Sharing has therefore allocated a MELD priority score of 22 for patients with HCC who meet the criteria detailed above. The score is increased every 3 months to reflect an additional 10% risk of mortality. This allocation policy requires continued analysis in order to make sure that patients with HCC are not being transplanted in favor of non-HCC patients or whether HCC patients are disadvantaged.

Although most liver transplant programs treat tumors in order to reduce the risk of tumor progression while on the waiting list, there are no controlled trials that support this practice.

There have been efforts to modestly expand the selection criteria for liver transplantation for HCC, and survival among patients with tumors that have been downstaged to fulfill the Milan criteria appears to be good.[24] Ultimately, tumor biology will likely define the outcome with liver transplantation and response to other treatment modalities.

TUMOR ABLATION

Ablative techniques (RFA and percutaneous ethanol ablation) are frequently used to treat small tumors by locally ablating the lesions percutaneously. In select patients, outcomes are similar to surgical resection; however, randomized controlled trials comparing these techniques to resection or liver transplantation have not been performed. A mathematical model comparing outcomes of these 2 modalities showed similar survival using a strategy of RFA followed by surgical resection in patients with tumor recurrence.[25]

RFA involves the local application of radiofrequency thermal energy to the lesion, thereby causing tumor necrosis. This approach was evaluated in a prospective study that included 86 consecutive patients with tumors ≤ 3 cm (the majority of whom were Child-Pugh class A with hepatitis C virus) who were treated with either PEI or RFA.[26] Complete tumor necrosis occurred more often following RFA (90% versus 80%), although results were not statistically significant. On average, fewer treatment sessions were required for RFA (1.2 versus 4.8). However, complications including bleeding, pleural effusions, cholecystitis, and hemobilia occurred more frequently with RFA (2% major and 8% minor complications for RFA versus none for the PEI group). Of concern is the potential for seeding along the needle track that has been reported in patients receiving RFA for solitary tumors. Based on this observation, RFA is often avoided for tumors that are adjacent to the hepatic capsule. In addition, tumor proximity to bile ducts and hepatic vessels may exclude some patients from this procedure.

TRANSARTERIAL CHEMOEMBOLIZATION

Disruption of the arterial blood supply and injection of chemotherapy (typically doxorubicin in combination with other agents) into hypervascular HCC lesions has been shown to prolong life.[27,28] **Patients with multifocal disease in the absence of portal vein invasion or CTP class C disease are typically eligible for this intervention.**

NOVEL SYSTEMIC CHEMOTHERAPY

The US Food and Drug Administration recently approved the Raf kinase and angiogenesis inhibitor sorafenib for treatment of advanced HCC in patients not eligible for the above treatments.[29] This study showed a modest survival benefit in patients receiving sorafenib compared to placebo, which is a landmark achievement because this is the first systemic agent to improve survival in patients with advanced HCC. Trials involving other targeted therapies alone or in combination are being performed.

ASSESSMENT OF RESPONSE TO TREATMENT

Cross-sectional imaging studies are typically used to survey patients for tumor recurrence or de novo tumor development following therapy for HCC. **Contrast-enhanced magnetic resonance imaging or computed tomography scans are typically performed every 3 to 6 months after therapy to survey for tumor recurrence.** Various standardized criteria are used to objectively assess response to therapies using radiographic criteria. The ideal system has yet to be determined, but there is a promising role for a more streamlined system that monitors response of the largest hepatic lesion.[30]

CONCLUSION

HCC is an aggressive tumor with a high case fatality rate. Successful treatment is contingent on early detection through widespread use of surveillance of patients at risk for HCC development. The future of treatment and early detection likely will be based on characterization of the molecular pathogenesis of this disease.

REFERENCES

1. Bosch FX, Ribes J, Diaz M, Cleries R. Primary liver cancer: worldwide incidence and trends. *Gastroenterology.* 2004;127:S5-S16.
2. Parkin DM. Global cancer statistics in the year 2000. *Lancet Oncol.* 2001;2:533-543.
3. El Serag HB, Mason AC. Rising incidence of hepatocellular carcinoma in the United States. *N Engl J Med.* 1999;340:745-750.
4. Sangiovanni A, Del Ninno E, Fasani P, et al. Increased survival of cirrhotic patients with a hepatocellular carcinoma detected during surveillance. *Gastroenterology.* 2004;126:1005-1014.
5. Zhang BH, Yang BH, Tang ZY. Randomized controlled trial of screening for hepatocellular carcinoma. *J Cancer Res Clin Oncol.* 2004;130:417-422.
6. El Serag HB, Siegel AB, Davila JA, et al. Treatment and outcomes of treating of hepatocellular carcinoma among Medicare recipients in the United States: a population-based study. *J Hepatol.* 2006;44:158-166.
7. Llovet JM, Bru C, Bruix J. Prognosis of hepatocellular carcinoma: the BCLC staging classification. *Semin Liver Dis.* 1999;19:329-338.
8. Okuda K, Ohtsuki T, Obata H, et al. Natural history of hepatocellular carcinoma and prognosis in relation to treatment. Study of 850 patients. *Cancer.* 1985;56:918-928.
9. Prospective validation of the CLIP score: a new prognostic system for patients with cirrhosis and hepatocellular carcinoma. The Cancer of the Liver Italian Program (CLIP) Investigators. *Hepatology.* 2000;31:840-845.
10. Bruix J, Llovet JM. Major achievements in hepatocellular carcinoma. *Lancet.* 2009;373:614-616.
11. Huo TI, Lin HC, Hsia CY, et al. The model for end-stage liver disease based cancer staging systems are better prognostic models for hepatocellular carcinoma: a prospective sequential survey. *Am J Gastroenterol.* 2007;102:1920-1930.
12. Marrero JA, Fontana RJ, Barrat A, et al. Prognosis of hepatocellular carcinoma: comparison of 7 staging systems in an American cohort. *Hepatology.* 2005;41:707-716.
13. Thorgeirsson SS, Lee JS, Grisham JW. Molecular prognostication of liver cancer: end of the beginning. *J Hepatol.* 2006;44:798-805.
14. Bruix J, Castells A, Bosch J, et al. Surgical resection of hepatocellular carcinoma in cirrhotic patients: prognostic value of preoperative portal pressure. *Gastroenterology.* 1996;111:1018-1022.

15. Ishizawa T, Hasegawa K, Aoki T, et al. Neither multiple tumors nor portal hypertension are surgical contraindications for hepatocellular carcinoma. *Gastroenterology.* 2008;134:1908-1916.

16. Takayama T, Makuuchi M, Hirohashi S, et al. Early hepatocellular carcinoma as an entity with a high rate of surgical cure. *Hepatology.* 1998;28:1241-1246.

17. Hoshida Y, Villanueva A, Kobayashi M, et al. Gene expression in fixed tissues and outcome in hepatocellular carcinoma. *N Engl J Med.* 2008;359:1995-2004.

18. Ji J, Shi J, Budhu A, et al. MicroRNA expression, survival, and response to interferon in liver cancer. *N Engl J Med.* 2009;361:1437-1447.

19. Lau WY, Leung TW, Ho SK, et al. Adjuvant intra-arterial iodine-131-labelled lipiodol for resectable hepatocellular carcinoma: a prospective randomised trial. *Lancet.* 1999;353:797-801.

20. Muto Y, Moriwaki H, Ninomiya M, et al. Prevention of second primary tumors by an acyclic retinoid, polyprenoic acid, in patients with hepatocellular carcinoma. Hepatoma Prevention Study Group. *N Engl J Med.* 1996;334:1561-1567.

21. Mazzaferro V, Regalia E, Doci R, et al. Liver transplantation for the treatment of small hepatocellular carcinomas in patients with cirrhosis. *N Engl J Med.* 1996;334:693-699.

22. Llovet JM, Bruix J, Fuster J, et al. Liver transplantation for small hepatocellular carcinoma: the tumor-node-metastasis classification does not have prognostic power. *Hepatology.* 1998;27:1572-1577.

23. Yao FY, Bass NM, Nikolai B, et al. Liver transplantation for hepatocellular carcinoma: analysis of survival according to the intention-to-treat principle and dropout from the waiting list. *Liver Transpl.* 2002;8:873-883.

24. Yao FY, Kerlan RK Jr, Hirose R, et al. Excellent outcome following down-staging of hepatocellular carcinoma prior to liver transplantation: an intention-to-treat analysis. *Hepatology.* 2008;48:819-827.

25. Cho YK, Kim JK, Kim WT, Chung JW. Hepatic resection versus radiofrequency ablation for very early stage hepatocellular carcinoma: a Markov model analysis. *Hepatology.* 2010;51:1284-1290.

26. Livraghi T, Goldberg SN, Lazzaroni S, Meloni F, Solbiati L, Gazelle GS. Small hepatocellular carcinoma: treatment with radio-frequency ablation versus ethanol injection. *Radiology.* 1999;210:655-661.

27. Llovet JM, Real MI, Montana X, et al. Arterial embolisation or chemoembolisation versus symptomatic treatment in patients with unresectable hepatocellular carcinoma: a randomised controlled trial. *Lancet.* 2002;359:1734-1739.

28. Lo CM, Ngan H, Tso WK, et al. Randomized controlled trial of transarterial lipiodol chemoembolization for unresectable hepatocellular carcinoma. *Hepatology.* 2002;35:1164-1171.

29. Llovet JM, Ricci S, Mazzaferro V, et al. Sorafenib in advanced hepatocellular carcinoma. *N Engl J Med.* 2008;359:378-390.

30. Riaz A, Miller FH, Kulik LM, et al. Imaging response in the primary index lesion and clinical outcomes following transarterial locoregional therapy for hepatocellular carcinoma. *JAMA.* 2010;303:1062-1069.

chapter

8

PULMONARY ISSUES IN PATIENTS WITH CIRRHOSIS

Michael F. Chang, MD, MSc

Cirrhosis is complicated by the development of pulmonary compromise in over 20% to 30% of individuals.[1] The main forms of pulmonary insult are divided between (1) pulmonary vascular compromise and (2) restrictive lung disease from compression by ascites or hydrothorax. Pulmonary vascular compromise occurs in 2 broad categories: intrapulmonary vascular dilatation (IPVD) characterized by the hepatopulmonary syndrome (HPS) and pulmonary artery vasoconstriction characterized by portopulmonary hypertension (POPH).

HEPATOPULMONARY SYNDROME

Background

HPS is a prevalent condition in patients with cirrhosis. HPS is estimated to affect anywhere between 5% and 32% of persons with advanced fibrosis; the variance is likely accounted for by different diagnostic thresholds.[2] HPS affects both men and women equally and is not associated with a particular etiology of liver disease or age at presentation. HPS has been rarely associated with acute liver injury and has been described in noncirrhotic portal hypertension. The condition is progressive, with median survival ranging from 11 to 41 months.[3]

HPS is defined by a constellation of findings, including (1) hypoxemia, (2) liver disease, and (3) IPVD. Based on the type of intrapulmonary shunting, HPS has been broken down into 2 types, type I and type II. Type I HPS is the

Zaman A. *Managing the Complications of Cirrhosis: A Practical Approach* (pp 97-110).

commonly referred to entity of HPS, where shunts occur at the precapillary and capillary level. Type II HPS refers to discrete pulmonary arteriovenous malformations (AVMs), which are diagnosed by angiography and can be managed with obliteration of the AVM. For the remainder of this section, we will be referring to type I HPS.

The mechanisms that lead to the dilatation of the pulmonary capillary bed and decreased arterial oxygenation are complex and only partially understood. Although the 3 components of the syndrome are key to making the diagnosis of this condition, the driving forces that impair oxygenation of blood in the pulmonary vasculature are dynamic and occur in 3 areas: shunting of blood through dilated capillaries, ventilation–perfusion (VQ) mismatch, and impaired diffusion of oxygen through alveolar capillary membranes.[1]

The shunting of blood through the pulmonary vasculature occurs due to the dilatation of the capillary and precapillary beds. Shunts related to discrete pulmonary AVMs and intracardiac shunts need to be distinguished between shunts related to type I HPS before the diagnosis can be certain. In HPS, there are 3 local mechanisms that act to impair oxygen exchange within the dilated vessel and 2 larger mechanisms that predispose to VQ mismatch.

The first local mechanism is an increase in blood flow rate related to splanchnic vasodilatation and increased cardiac output, decreasing the time for gas exchange. Increases in cardiac demand and output (ie, exertion) result in worsening hypoxia due to the further increases in blood flow rate and decreased transit time in the pulmonary vascular bed. The second mechanism contributing to hypoxemia is dilatation of the capillaries and reduced oxygen diffusion to the center of the blood vessel. Based on laminar flow dynamics, erythrocytes (ie, hemoglobin) concentrate at the center of the capillary where there is the highest flow rate, the shortest exposure time for gas exchange, and the least oxygen tension. The third mechanism is the formation of direct capillary shunts that completely bypass the alveoli and present deoxygenated blood to the pulmonary capillary veins.[3] An important observation in this setting is that type I HPS improves with 100% oxygen inspiration, suggesting that increased oxygen concentration at the alveolar level improves diffusion into the dilated capillaries. True shunts (intracardiac and pulmonary AVMs) do not respond to inspiration of 100% oxygen, because the shunted blood is never exposed to the enriched oxygen. Patients with HPS universally have an abnormal diffusion capacity for carbon monoxide, based on pulmonary function testing. Clinically, patients with HPS improve with oxygen supplementation, though the effect on survival is unknown.[1]

Within the lung itself, 2 other mechanisms have been noted that contribute to hypoxemia, predominantly through mechanisms which favor VQ mismatch. Normal pulmonary vascular response to hypoxemia will result in increased arteriolar tone in the hypoxic segment, forcing blood to segments with better ventilation. This response is attenuated in patients with cirrhosis, thus allowing hypoxic segments to remain perfused. The second process that contributes to VQ mismatch is related to loss of vascular tone in the pulmonary vessels. The diminished arteriolar tone does not accommodate gravitational blood flow changes, resulting in an inability to prevent vascular pooling at the lung bases, leading to a drop in oxygen saturation > 5% when moving from a supine position to a sitting position (orthodeoxia) and increased shortness of breath (platypnea).[4]

Multiple mechanisms have been suggested to explain the vascular changes seen in HPS. A detailed discussion of the mechanisms is beyond the scope of this chapter. The predominant theories behind the mechanisms that lead to vascular dilatation are believed to be mediated by nitric oxide, either from increased production or decreased breakdown.

Diagnosis

The dominant pathophysiologic mechanism leading to HPS is dilatation of the pulmonary capillary bed. The normal range in capillary diameter in the lung is 8 to 15 μm. In the setting of HPS, capillaries are dilated to 15 to 100 μm. Symptoms associated with HPS include dyspnea on exertion (DOE), hypoxemia when moving from a supine to a sitting position (orthodeoxia), and shortness of breath when moving from a supine to a sitting position (platypnea). **The presentation of hypoxia, as seen on routine pulse oximetry on room air with a value below 94%, in a patient with liver disease should be further investigated with an arterial blood gas (ABG) measurement. The presence of an alveolar-arterial oxygen gradient > 15 mm Hg and a partial pressure of oxygen ≤ 80 mm Hg suggests the presence of HPS.** If HPS is suspected after the initial ABG, a repeat ABG should be considered on 100% oxygen via nonrebreather face mask. An arterial partial pressure of oxygen (PaO_2) under 300 mm Hg after breathing several minutes of 100% oxygen should raise concerns for severe HPS, discrete AVMs, or an intracardiac shunt. Hypoxemia related to intracardiac shunts and pulmonary AVMs does not respond to inspiration of 100% oxygen. **The diagnosis of HPS is confirmed with a contrast-enhanced transthoracic echocardiogram, also known as a *bubble study*.** A contrast echocardiogram is performed with agitated saline injected into a peripheral vein. Agitation of saline produces microbubbles that are 10 to 90 μm in diameter; in the normal lung, these microbubbles are trapped in the pulmonary capillary bed and absorbed. In patients with HPS, pulmonary capillary dilatations allow rapid passage of the microbubbles from the pulmonary arterial side to the pulmonary venous side. The presentation of microbubbles in the left atrium between 3 to 6 heartbeats after injection of the agitated saline suggests the presence of a pulmonary shunt. Microbubbles that present within 1 to 3 heartbeats in the left atrium suggest an intracardiac shunt (Table 8-1).[3]

The use of a technetium-labeled macroaggregated albumin (^{99m}Tc-MAA) lung scan allows for a quantitative measurement of pulmonary shunting.

Table 8-1

Evaluation of Hepatopulmonary Syndrome

Clinical Objective	Findings		Discussion
Symptoms	DOE, orthodeoxia, platypnea		
Physical exam	Nonspecific		Spider nevi, digital clubbing, acrocyanosis
Pulse oximetry on room air	Values < 94% on room air should be followed up with an arterial blood gas to measure arterial oxygen concentration and A-a gradient		
ABG on room air	A-a gradient ≥ 15 mm Hg	80 mm Hg ≤ PaO_2	Mild
		60 ≤ PaO_2 < 80	Moderate
		50 ≤ PaO_2 < 60	Severe
		PaO_2 < 50	Very severe
ABG on 100% O_2	A-a gradient ≥ 15 mm HG + PaO_2 < 300 mm Hg		Consider severe HPS, AVMs, or intracardiac shunt
Contrast echo (bubble study)	Agitated saline creates microbubbles 10 to 90 μm in diameter that are injected into a peripheral vein		Presence of bubbles in the left atrium after 3 heartbeats suggests HPS
99mTc-MAA lung perfusion scan	99mTc-MAA molecules are 20 to 90 μm in diameter and are injected into a peripheral vein		> 6% shunt fraction suggests HPS; > 20% suggests very severe HPS

DOE indicates dyspnea on exertion; A-a gradient, alveolar-arterial oxygen gradient; ABG, arterial blood gas; HPS, hepatopulmonary syndrome; AVM, arteriovenous malformation; 99mTc-MAA, technetium-labeled macroaggregated albumin

This test utilizes radioactive-labeled large molecules of aggregated albumin, which measure from 20 to 90 μm in diameter. Similar to the saline microbubbles, the macroaggregated albumin can escape the pulmonary capillary bed in the presence of HPS and be detected in the brain and kidneys. The shunt fraction can be calculated based on the scintigraphic analysis of distribution of radioactivity; a brain fraction ≥ 6% is highly suggestive of HPS. This study is less sensitive and more invasive than contrast echocardiography and should be performed only when the additional prognostic information is required. Pulmonary AVMs and intracardiac shunts can present false-positive tests, so caution should be exercised and evaluation for these entities should be considered.

Treatment

Liver transplantation remains the only proven therapy for HPS.
Small intervention studies of antibiotics, tumor necrosis factor (TNF)-alpha
inhibitors, inhaled nitric oxide, nitric oxide inhibitors, steroids, beta blockers,
and vascular shunts have all proven to be ineffective or even harmful.[1] At this
time, the diagnosis of severe HPS (alveolar-arterial (A-a) gradient ≥ 15 mm Hg,
50 ≤ PaO_2 < 60 mm Hg) is a strong primary indicator for liver transplantation, even in the setting of good liver function. Unfortunately, with very severe
HPS (A-a gradient ≥ 15 mm Hg, PaO_2 < 50 mm Hg or [99mTc]-MAA shunt
> 20%), liver transplantation is contraindicated due to high perioperative mor-
tality. **Patients with mild, moderate, or severe HPS should be referred
for liver transplant evaluation, because the natural history of HPS
suggests a decrease of PaO_2 of 5 to 10 mm Hg per year, which can
result in disqualification from liver transplant if very severe HPS
develops.**[5]

Alternatives

Use of supplemental oxygen is recommended for symptomatic management
of HPS. No other alternative therapies are available at this time except liver
transplantation.

Referral

Patients with documented HPS should be referred for a liver transplant
evaluation. In the largest series of patients transplanted for HPS at the Mayo
Clinic, 5-year survival was found to be 76%, which is similar to results from
liver transplantation related to other disease conditions. Conversely, survival without transplantation was universally poor, with only 26% survival at
5 years. Given that the evaluation process for liver transplantation can be rigorous and the social, financial, and substance use requirements be strict, early
referral provides the best chance at being listed for liver transplantation. Only
patients with severe HPS qualify for priority on the liver transplant waiting list
(exception points).[3]

PORTOPULMONARY HYPERTENSION

Background

POPH is a condition that describes the constellation of pulmonary artery
hypertension in the setting of portal hypertension, with or without significant
liver disease.[6] This condition is generally underrecognized, because the presenting symptom of DOE and fatigue is often masked by multiple comorbid
conditions in the setting of advanced liver disease. Large population studies

have not been conducted to identify the exact prevalence of this condition in patients with cirrhosis. In select populations of persons referred for liver transplantation, up to 5% have been found to have POPH. The condition appears to occur slightly more commonly in women compared to men, presents usually in the fifth decade of life, and is independent from the severity of liver disease.[6] Overall survival is poor in advanced POPH without treatment, with a 1-year mortality of over 50%.[7]

The pathogenesis of POPH is poorly understood. Histological evaluation reveals proliferative pulmonary arteriopathy with formation of plexiform lesions, necrotizing arteritis with fibrinoid necrosis, and thrombosis.[1] Sheer stress in the arteriolar wall from increased cardiac output is believed to be the inciting event, leading to a cascade response that is catalyzed by potent vasoconstrictors escaping from the liver and attenuated compensatory mechanisms in the pulmonary vascular bed. Forces favoring vascular constriction include the escape of vasoactive substances and bacterial endotoxin within hepatic portosystemic shunts and decreased metabolism of endothelin-1 and serotonin, which are both potent vasoconstrictors. Decreases in prostacyclin and nitric oxide production, both potent vasodilators, promulgate the pulmonary hypertension via the loss of vasodilatory pathways. Prolonged injury and inflammation lead to organized fibrosis, remodeling, and proliferation of the vascular bed.[8]

Diagnosis

The diagnosis of POPH requires a high index of suspicion prompted by history and physical exam. DOE in the patient with portal hypertension should be evaluated and the differential diagnosis carefully considered. The presence of hypoxia by pulse oximetry should prompt consideration for HPS, chronic obstructive pulmonary disease in the alcoholic, or underlying cardiopulmonary conditions. **Likewise, new dyspnea or rapidly worsening dyspnea should prompt consideration of POPH.**[9] Physical exam evidence of right heart strain or failure with an audible S3, tricuspid murmur, split P2, right ventricular heave, and peripheral edema on exam should prompt further investigation. An electrocardiogram (EKG) that demonstrates right heart strain, new right bundle branch block, or right axis deviation and a chest x-ray with findings of prominent pulmonary arteries, vascular pruning, and cardiomegaly are nonspecific but suggestive findings. **Suspicion for pulmonary hypertension should be followed up with an echocardiogram. Identification of a pulmonary artery systolic pressure of 50 mm Hg or more should prompt cardiac catheterization for a more definitive evaluation.** In up to 20% to 30% of patients referred for a cardiac echo, estimates of right heart pressure will not be possible, due to the absence of tricuspid regurgitation, which is necessary to estimate right heart pressure. In these situations, clinical evidence and EKG evidence of right heart strain in the absence of tricuspid regurgitation will need to be considered to determine the need for further testing (Figure 8-1).[10]

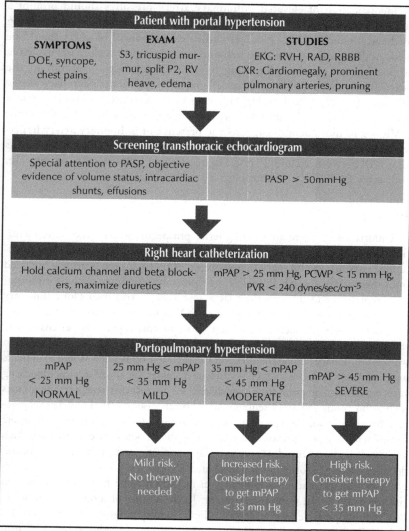

Figure 8-1. Algorithm to diagnose portopulmonary hypertension. DOE indicates dyspnea on exertion; RV, right ventricular; EKG, electrocardiogram; RVH, right ventricular hypertrophy; RBBB, right bundle branch block; CXR, chest X-ray; PASP, pulmonary artery systolic pressure; mPAP, mean pulmonary artery pressure; PCWP, pulmonary capillary wedge pressure; PVR, pulmonary vascular resistance; RAD, right axis deviation.

Identification of elevated pulmonary artery pressures should prompt a right heart catheterization. Prior to cardiac catheterization, confounding medications such as beta blockers and calcium channel blockers should be held. Additionally, volume status should be maintained as close to euvolemia as possible, to avoid confounding by elevated left-sided pressures in the heart. In the absence of high left-sided pressures (pulmonary capillary wedge pressure [PCWP] < 15 mm Hg), identification of a mean pulmonary artery pressure (mPAP) > 25 mm Hg with high pulmonary vascular resistance (PVR > 240 dyne/s/cm^{-5}) suggests the presence of pulmonary artery hypertension. Staging of POPH is based on the mPAP. Mild POPH is defined as an mPAP between 25 and 35 mm Hg, moderate POPH as 36 to 45 mm Hg, and severe POPH as > 45 mm Hg.[6]

Treatment

Unfortunately, there are no long-term, prospective studies that have identified the optimal management of POPH. In fact, within the larger trials of medications to control pulmonary hypertension, POPH has been routinely excluded from these trials, though POPH is the third most common reason for pulmonary hypertension.[11] Despite these facts, several of the treatments for pulmonary artery hypertension have been applied to POPH with reasonable results.

Calcium channel blockers have been shown to worsen portal hypertension and should be avoided in this condition. Additionally, propranolol has been shown to worsen pulmonary hemodynamics and should likely be avoided as well in patients with moderate to severe POPH.[12] Current therapies are aimed at either blocking vasoconstriction or promoting vasodilatation. Endothelin receptor antagonists such as bosentan and ambrisentan work to block vasoconstriction, whereas prostacyclin analogs such as epoprostenol, treprostinil, and iloprost work to promote vasodilatation. Another class of medications, phosphodiesterase-5 inhibitors such as sildenafil, promotes pulmonary vascular vasodilatation by inhibiting the breakdown of cyclic guanosine monophosphate (GMP).[6]

Liver transplantation is indicated in mild POPH with minimal increased risk for death at the time of transplant. In the setting of moderate and severe POPH, perioperative liver transplantation mortality ranges from 60% to 100% if the mPAP cannot be controlled with medication and reduced below 35 mm Hg. **Current recommendations by the American Association for the Study of Liver Diseases provide for liver transplant priority in the setting of moderate to severe POPH, provided that the mPAP can be reduced below 35 mm Hg and the PVR below 400 dyne/s/cm^{-5}.**[13]

Alternatives

There are no alternative therapies to the above-described treatment options. Mortality at 1 year is very high in the absence of therapy.

Referral

Given the high mortality associated with moderate to severe POPH, referral to a liver transplant center with expertise in the management of patients with portal hypertension and POPH is recommended. Given that median survival without therapy is 6 months, delays in referral and management should be avoided.[14]

HEPATIC HYDROTHORAX

Background

Hepatic hydrothorax is the development of a pleural effusion in the background of portal hypertension and the absence of a primary cardiac, pulmonary, or oncologic etiology. This entity is seen in up to 10% of patients with advanced cirrhosis and almost always in the presence of abdominal ascites. Cases of isolated hepatic hydrothorax comprise less than 10% of patients presenting with this complication of portal hypertension.[15]

The etiology of hepatic hydrothorax is believed to be secondary to passage of peritoneal fluid through small defects in the diaphragm. Due to the negative intrathoracic pressure, fluid preferentially moves into the pleural space from the peritoneal cavity. Multiple elegant studies have demonstrated this unidirectional movement using a wide range of markers injected into the abdomen, from carbon dioxide to methylene blue to radioactive isotopes.[16]

The most plausible explanation to date describes small herniations of the peritoneum through gaps in the collagen bundles at the tendinous portion of the diaphragm. These herniations rupture, producing small connections between the peritoneal and pleural space, allowing passage of fluid. The right-sided preference of the effusion is attributed to the weaker, less muscular right diaphragm.[15] Overall, 85% of hepatic hydrothoraces present with isolated right-sided effusion, 13% with isolated left-sided effusion, and 2% with bilateral effusions.[17]

Diagnosis

The most common presentation of hepatic hydrothorax is shortness of breath due to loss of lung volume and an isolated right-sided effusion. Patients presenting with progressive dyspnea should undergo a routine evaluation that involves a thorough history and physical exam, as well as routine lab work, which should include a complete blood count, chemistries, and liver function tests. Consideration of primary pulmonary and cardiac etiologies should be ruled out, as well as anemia from gastrointestinal bleeding. Physical exam will invariably identify a large pleural effusion based on decreased breath sounds, dullness to percussion, decreased tactile fremitus,

Treatment

Given the relationship of hepatic hydrothorax to ascites, medical management has focused on the management of ascites. Sodium restriction is the cornerstone of therapy, because any medical intervention will fail in the setting of patient noncompliance. An attempt at restricting sodium to < 2000 mg per day is recommended (equivalent to 90 mEq/day of sodium). Spironolactone is the preferred diuretic due to its potency in patients with cirrhosis, although a balanced use of furosemide and spironolactone is most common. Under maximal medical therapy, if a patient continues to require more than one thoracentesis every 2 to 3 weeks, alternative therapies should be evaluated (Figure 8-2). Given that hepatic hydrothorax often occurs late in the course of liver disease, liver transplantation should be considered.[16]

Alternatives

If maximal medical therapy fails and patient noncompliance has been addressed, alternative therapies for hepatic hydrothorax should be considered. Within the literature, several options for management have been described, none of which have been studied in a controlled, randomized study. Given the very low incidence of this condition, prospective intervention studies for hepatic hydrothorax are unlikely in the future. Repeated thoracentesis runs the risk of causing bleeding, infection, and pneumothorax.[17] **Pleurodesis is rarely effective due to the inability to keep the pleural space coapted long enough for adhesion to occur and is often complicated by fever, loculations, and infection.[18] The long-term placement of a chest tube is strongly discouraged due to high associated morbidity and mortality.[19]** Use of video-assisted thoroscopy to repair disruptions in the diaphragm has been described, though reports are limited and success rates variable, suggesting that this therapy should be pursued only in centers with experience with these procedures or in palliative cases.[18,20]

The use of a transjugular intrahepatic portosystemic shunt (TIPS) has been the most widely described intervention for the treatment of hepatic hydrothorax, though no comparative efficacy trials exist for this intervention. TIPS has been shown to improve refractory hydrothorax in up to 70% of patients. Unfortunately, this procedure is complicated by portosystemic encephalopathy in 30% of patients and is limited to patients with relatively intact liver function. Patients with a bilirubin < 3 mg/dL, age < 65, and no history of encephalopathy are the best candidates for this intervention.[21,22] Likewise, patients with a model for end-stage liver disease (MELD) score > 15 have almost twice the risk of dying compared to those with a MELD score < 15.[23] Ultimately, TIPS is a viable treatment option for hepatic hydrothorax in select populations; however, liver transplantation is the definitive treatment to address hepatic dysfunction and portal hypertension leading to the formation of ascites and hydrothorax. Hepatic hydrothorax

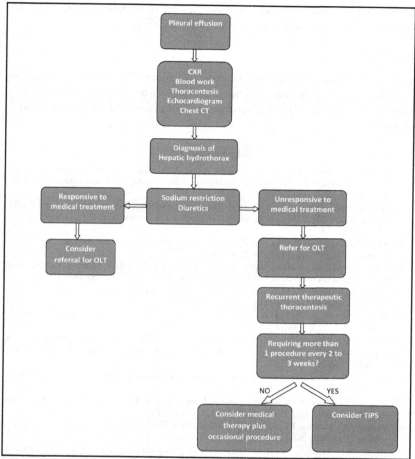

Figure 8-2. Evaluation of pleural effusion in cirrhosis.

and egophony (E-to-A change). Effusions < 300 cc are difficult to detect by physical exam. The extent of the effusion can be revealed by chest x-ray. Once identified, a thoracentesis is necessary to characterize the fluid. Up to 30% of persons presenting with new effusions and known ascites do not have hepatic hydrothorax.[16] Initial observation of the fluid for color, character, and odor is helpful in identifying blood, infection, biliary fluid, or transudate. **Pleural fluid should be sent for cell count, cytology, and chemical analysis, which should include the following: protein, albumin, lactate dehydrogenase (LDH), cholesterol, glucose, and amylase.** In those presenting with an isolated right-sided effusion without prior history of ascites, an echocardiogram is indicated to further rule out a cardiac source for the effusion.[15]

has not been shown to worsen outcomes in liver transplant, and patients may be able to obtain transplant priority through their regional review board.[24]

Referral

Given the strong association between the presence of hepatic hydrothorax and advanced liver disease, patients presenting with this condition should be referred for specialty care by a hepatologist and considered for liver transplant evaluation.

REFERENCES

1. Rodríguez-Roisin R, Krowka MJ, Hervé P, Fallon MB; ERS Task Force Pulmonary-Hepatic Vascular Disorders (PHD) Scientific Committee. Pulmonary-hepatic vascular disorders (PHD). *Eur Respir J.* 2004;24:861-880.

2. Schenk P, Fuhrmann V, Madl C, et al. Hepatopulmonary syndrome: prevalence and predictive value of various cut offs for arterial oxygenation and their clinical consequences. *Gut.* 2002;51:853-859.

3. Rodriguez-Roisin R, Krowka MJ. Hepatopulmonary syndrome—a liver-induced lung vascular disorder. *N Engl J Med.* 2008;358:2378-2387.

4. Gómez FP, Martínez-Pallí G, Barberà JA, Roca J, Navasa M, Rodríguez-Roisin R. Gas exchange mechanism of orthodeoxia in hepatopulmonary syndrome. *Hepatology.* 2004;40:660-666.

5. Swanson KL, Wiesner RH, Krowka MJ. Natural history of hepatopulmonary syndrome: impact of liver transplantation. *Hepatology.* 2005;41:1122-1129.

6. Stauber RE, Olschewski H. Portopulmonary hypertension: short review. *Eur J Gastroenterol Hepatol.* 2010;22:385-389.

7. Swanson KL, Wiesner RH, Nyberg SL, Rosen CB, Krowka MJ. Survival in portopulmonary hypertension: Mayo Clinic experience categorized by treatment subgroups. *Am J Transplant.* 2008;8:2445-2453.

8. Porres-Aguilar M, Zuckerman MJ, Figueroa-Casas JB, Krowka MJ. Portopulmonary hypertension: state of the art. *Ann Hepatol.* 2008;7:321-330.

9. Swanson KL, Krowka MJ. Screen for portopulmonary hypertension, especially in liver transplant candidates. *Cleve Clin J Med.* 2008;75:121-122,125-130,133.

10. Krowka MJ, Swanson KL, Frantz RP, McGoon MD, Wiesner RH. Portopulmonary hypertension: results from a 10-year screening algorithm. *Hepatology.* 2006;44:1502-1510.

11. Krowka MJ, Swanson KL. How should we treat portopulmonary hypertension? *Eur Respir J.* 2006;28:466-467.

12. Provencher S, Herve P, Jais X, et al. Deleterious effects of beta-blockers on exercise capacity and hemodynamics in patients with portopulmonary hypertension. *Gastroenterology.* 2006;130:120-126.

13. Krowka MJ, Fallon MB, Mulligan DC, Gish RG. Model for end-stage liver disease (MELD) exception for portopulmonary hypertension. *Liver Transpl.* 2006;12(12 Suppl 3):S114-S116.

14. Robalino BD, Moodie DS. Association between primary pulmonary hypertension and portal hypertension: analysis of its pathophysiology and clinical, laboratory and hemodynamic manifestations. *J Am Coll Cardiol.* 1991;17:492-498.

15. Roussos A, Philippou N, Mantzaris GJ, Gourgouliannis KI. Hepatic hydrothorax: pathophysiology diagnosis and management. *J Gastroenterol Hepatol.* 2007;22:1388-1393.

16. Kiafar C, Gilani N. Hepatic hydrothorax: current concepts of pathophysiology and treatment options. *Ann Hepatol.* 2008;7:313-320.

17. Lazaridis KN, Frank JW, Krowka MJ, Kamath PS. Hepatic hydrothorax: pathogenesis, diagnosis, and management. *Am J Med.* 1999;107:262-267.

18. Milanez de Campos JR, Filho LO, de Campos Werebe E, et al. Thoracoscopy and talc poudrage in the management of hepatic hydrothorax. *Chest.* 2000;118:13-17.

19. Orman ES, Lok AS. Outcomes of patients with chest tube insertion for hepatic hydrothorax. *Hepatol Int.* 2009;3:582-586.
20. Cerfolio RJ, Bryant AS. Efficacy of video-assisted thoracoscopic surgery with talc pleurodesis for porous diaphragm syndrome in patients with refractory hepatic hydrothorax. *Ann Thorac Surg.* 2006;82:457-459.
21. Rossle M, Gerbes AL. TIPS for the treatment of refractory ascites, hepatorenal syndrome and hepatic hydrothorax: a critical update. *Gut.* 2010;59:988-1000.
22. Gerbes AL, Gulberg V. Benefit of TIPS for patients with refractory or recidivant ascites: serum bilirubin may make the difference. *Hepatology.* 2005;41:217.
23. Dhanasekaran R, West JK, Gonzales PC, et al. Transjugular intrahepatic portosystemic shunt for symptomatic refractory hepatic hydrothorax in patients with cirrhosis. *Am J Gastroenterol.* 2010;105:635-641.
24. Serste T, Moreno C, Francoz C, et al. The impact of preoperative hepatic hydrothorax on the outcome of adult liver transplantation. *Eur J Gastroenterol Hepatol.* 2010;22:207-212.

PREOPERATIVE RISK ASSESSMENT IN PATIENTS WITH CIRRHOSIS

Atif Zaman, MD, MPH and Kenneth Ingram, PA-C

Cirrhosis of the liver is a final common pathway for all chronic liver diseases; it is defined as progressive disease of the liver characterized by diffuse damage to hepatic parenchymal cells with nodular degeneration, fibrosis, and disturbance of normal architecture.[1] Cirrhosis occurs worldwide in both genders regardless of age or race.[2] Epidemiologic data are limited, partially because of delays in diagnosis; up to 40% of individuals with cirrhosis are asymptomatic.[3] Data reporting methods that utilize death certificate reporting are also likely to underrepresent the true prevalence and impact of cirrhosis and chronic liver diseases due to the use of a primary cause of death, which frequently lists complications related to cirrhosis but do not explicitly contain the diagnosis of cirrhosis and thus cause underestimation of the true impact of cirrhosis.[4] In 2001, cirrhosis was the sixth leading cause of death among adults in developed countries and is increasing worldwide.[2] In 1998, cirrhosis was responsible for approximately 45,000 deaths and was the at least the 10th and possibly as high as the eighth leading cause of death in the United States based on mortality data.[5] Cirrhosis, including unrecognized disease with well-compensated hepatic function, is not uncommon and is estimated to be present in 1% of the population worldwide.[6]

SURGERY IN PATIENTS WITH LIVER DISEASE

Patients with liver disease frequently undergo surgery. Among patients with advanced liver disease, up to 10% will undergo an operation during the last

Zaman A. *Managing the Complications of Cirrhosis: A Practical Approach* (pp 111-124).

2 years of life.[7] Surgery other than liver transplantation in patients with underlying liver disease has an impact on outcomes, including morbidity and mortality.[8] Liver enzyme elevation frequently occurs in patients postoperatively.[9] Individuals with mild chronic liver disease with preserved hepatic clearance and synthetic function who do not have evidence of portal hypertension may undergo elective surgery with good outcomes.[10,11] Patients with cirrhosis are at risk of severe hepatic decompensation. A variety of factors contribute to the increased risks of patients with cirrhosis undergoing surgical procedures; variations in circulation including decreased systemic vascular resistance and increased cardiac output related to hyperdynamic circulation may lead to decreased hepatic perfusion of the cirrhotic liver at baseline. The type of anesthesia used, bleeding, hypotension, mechanical ventilation, vasoactive drugs, and pneumoperitoneum during laparoscopic procedures may all contribute to further decreases in blood flow during surgery.[12,13] Patients with cirrhosis are also at risk of hypoxemia perioperatively; risk factors include ascites, hepatic hydrothorax, aspiration, or underlying hepatopulmonary syndrome or portopulmonary hypertension, both of which significantly increase perioperative mortality.[12]

PREOPERATIVE EVALUATION

A careful preoperative assessment for the presence of underlying liver disease is of paramount importance when surgery is being considered. This evaluation is of increased importance in patients undergoing elective surgical procedures so that patients with contraindications can be identified and care for those with potentially modifiable risk factors can be optimized to improve outcomes. The goal is to identify the existence of underlying liver disease utilizing the least invasive means possible.[8] As previously mentioned, liver disease including cirrhosis is frequently asymptomatic, and a thorough history and physical examination can uncover important clues that may dramatically alter patient management. A focused history for risk factors of underlying liver disease should include questions regarding symptoms such as persistent fatigue, itching, or jaundice. Specific risk factors for viral hepatitis and other chronic liver diseases such as blood transfusions or other blood products prior to 1992, history of injection or intranasal drug use, obesity, diabetes, dyslipidemia, as well as amount and duration of alcohol use should be reviewed. A history of unexplained bleeding, bruising, muscle wasting, or gastrointestinal bleeding should prompt further evaluation. A family history of liver disease and jaundice should also be explored. Physical exam findings associated with liver disease include cirrhosis, temporal or thenar muscle wasting, gynecomatia, hypogonadism, hepatomegaly, or smaller than expected liver span with firm nodular liver surface, ascites, asterixis, spider hemangioma, jaundice, white nails, Dupuytren's contracture, caput medusa, or fetor hepaticus.

If the history and physical examination are not concerning for evidence of underlying liver disease, the role of routine laboratory evaluation of liver biochemistries is debatable. Hanje and Patel[8] and Malik and Ahmad[14] do not recommend routine testing based on the results of a study of 7620 preoperative patients that identified only 11 patients with abnormal liver function tests prior to elective surgery.[15] O'Leary et al[12] also stopped short of recommending routine preoperative liver function testing but pointed out that the prevalence of abnormal serum aminotransferases in the adult US population is 9.8%,[16] and these elevations may be indicative of underlying liver disease but may also be associated with increased risk of coronary heart disease due to association with metabolic syndrome.[17] If history and physical examination are not suggestive of liver disease, it is acceptable to proceed with elective surgery without further workup.

EVALUATION OF THE PATIENT WITH EVIDENCE OF LIVER DISEASE

If pre-existing liver disease is present or suspected, particularly if clinical evidence is suggestive of underlying cirrhosis, further preoperative workup is warranted (Table 9-1). Initial testing should include a complete metabolic panel, including serum aminotransferases (aspartate aminotransferase [AST]/alanine aminotransferase [ALT]), alkaline phosphatase, total bilirubin, and albumin levels. Blood counts including hemoglobin, white blood cells, and platelet count as well as a prothrombin time–internationalized ratio (PT-INR) may also provide important clues regarding the severity of any underlying hepatic abnormalities. Additionally, disease-specific evaluation for common etiologies of liver disease should be considered, including serologic markers of viral hepatitis, autoimmune liver disease, primary biliary cirrhosis, hemochromatosis, Wilson's disease, and alpha-1-antitrypsin deficiency. Abdominal imaging with ultrasound, computed tomography (CT), or magnetic resonance imaging (MRI) is useful to identify hepatic lesions, ascites, or evidence of overt cirrhosis and portal hypertension such as the presence of gastric varices or splenomegaly. **It is valuable to remember that although overt cirrhosis and portal hypertension can be detected by abdominal imaging, the lack of findings associated with portal hypertension does not exclude the presence of cirrhosis or undetected portal hypertension, and liver biopsy currently remains the gold standard for the diagnosis and staging of liver disease.[12]**

SURGERY IN THE PATIENT WITH LIVER DISEASE

Surgery in the patient with known liver disease can be roughly divided into 2 categories: elective and emergent. In the case of elective operations,

Table 9-1

Components of Preoperative Assessment of Hepatic Function in Patients With Existing Liver Disease

- Chemistry
  - □ Albumin
    - ◆ Marker of synthetic function
  - □ Total bilirubin
    - ◆ Marker of clearance function
  - □ Creatinine
    - ◆ Estimate of renal function
    - ◆ May overestimate renal function in muscle wasting
- Hematology
  - □ White blood cells, red blood cells, platelets
    - ◆ Pancytopenia common in cirrhosis
    - ◆ Thyrombocytopenia is a surrogate for portal hypertension
  - □ INR
    - ◆ Marker of hepatic synthetic function
- Imaging
  - □ Ultrasound or CT of abdomen
    - ◆ Evaluate for evidence of cirrhosis and/or portal hypertension
    - ◆ Ascites, splenomegaly, shrunken/nodular liver, enlarged portal vein
- Physical exam findings suggestive of cirrhosis
  - □ Temporal or thenar muscle wasting
  - □ Jaundice
  - □ Smaller than expected liver span/firm nodular liver surface
  - □ Splenomegaly
  - □ Ascites
  - □ Spider hemangioma
  - □ Fetor hepaticus

INR indicates international normalized ratio; CT, computed tomography

some contraindications to operative procedures in patients with liver disease have been identified (Table 9-2) and include acute liver failure, defined as the acute onset of coagulopathy and hepatic encephalopathy with an onset of < 26 weeks in a patient without pre-existing liver disease; acute viral hepatitis; and alcoholic hepatitis.[18-20] Acute liver injury may also be caused by drugs and hepatotoxins, including prescription and over-the-counter medications, herbal and other natural supplements, as well as some types of wild mushrooms. All types of acute hepatitis carry an increased operative risk.[21] The increased risks in patients with acute hepatitis are likely a result of hepatic dysfunction

— Table 9-2 —

Contraindications to Elective Surgery Due to Acute Liver Injury Reassessment After Resolution

- Alcoholic hepatitis
  - □ Common presentation: right upper quadrant pain, jaundice, fever, elevated liver enzymes, leukocytosis, and gallbladder wall thickening due to hypoalbuminemia
  - □ May be mistaken as acute cholecystitis or ascending cholangitis with disastrous outcome
- Acute liver failure
  - □ Acute coagulopathy and hepatic encephalopathy < 26 weeks without previous liver disease
- Acute viral hepatitis
- Acute hepatotoxicity
  - □ Prescription medications
  - □ Over-the-counter medications and herbal supplements
  - □ Some wild mushrooms

— Table 9-3 —

General Contraindications to Elective Surgery in Patients With Liver Disease

- Severe uncorrectable coagulopathy
- Acute renal failure
- Hypoxemia
- Serum bilirubin > 11 mg/dL
- Cardiomyopathy

that is associated with acute hepatocellular injury. Fortunately, most cases of acute hepatitis are self-limited and consideration of surgery can be reassessed once resolution has occurred and the patient has returned to baseline. Other contraindications to elective surgery in patients with liver disease include severe uncorrectable coagulopathy, acute renal failure, hypoxemia, serum bilirubin > 11 mg/dL, and cardiomyopathy (Table 9-3).

Special emphasis is warranted in the case of acute alcoholic hepatitis. **Common presentations of alcoholic hepatitis can include right upper quadrant abdominal pain, jaundice, fever, elevated liver function tests, and leukocytosis. This presentation must be distinguished**

from acute cholecystitis and ascending cholangitis.[22] The clinical picture may be further confused by gallbladder wall edema related to hypoalbuminemia, which may be present in alcoholic hepatitis due to poor nutritional status or decreased hepatic synthetic function in the case of underlying cirrhosis with superimposed acute on chronic alcoholic hepatitis. Distinguishing alcoholic hepatitis from an acute biliary process is vital due to the increased operative risk noted in patients with alcoholic hepatitis. A retrospective case series comparing laparoscopic and percutaneous liver biopsy in 51 patients with alcoholic liver disease resulted in 58% versus 10% mortality, respectively.[20] Only one death was related to intra-abdominal hemorrhage in the laparoscopic group and thus the increased mortality was associated with abdominal surgery rather than risks associated with liver biopsy.

Surgery may proceed in asymptomatic patients with known mild to moderate chronic liver disease in the presence of an imaging study that does not demonstrate a cirrhotic-appearing liver and/or evidence of portal hypertension and normal or mildly elevated AST/ALT, < 3 times the upper limit of normal, combined with normal markers of hepatic synthetic and clearance function; albumin and PT-INR, and total bilirubin, respectively, along with normal platelets.[11,23] Further risk assessment is required, even in the case of normal aminotransferases in patients with synthetic or clearance dysfunction as well as those with decreased platelet counts. The presence of thrombocytopenia is a surrogate marker for possible portal hypertension.

ASSESSMENT OF SURGICAL RISK IN THE CIRRHOTIC PATIENT

Data from the Nationwide Inpatient Sample database compared nearly 23,000 elective abdominal and cardiovascular surgeries between 1998 and 2005 in patients with cirrhosis of the liver, with or without portal hypertension, with 2.8 million noncirrhotic patients. Patients with cirrhosis experience significantly higher in-hospital mortality, increased lengths of stay, and higher total hospital charges.[24] This study cautioned that most operations on patients with cirrhosis were undertaken at large urban centers, many of which are academic centers with considerable experience in cirrhotic patients and transplant programs; outcomes in less experienced centers may differ.

Thoughtful selection in the patient with cirrhosis who is being considered for a surgical procedure is the foundation upon which optimal outcomes are built upon. The best method for stratifying surgical patients has yet to be determined. In a recent editorial, Henderson[25] reminded us that in the context of surgery, "there is no such thing as a good cirrhotic patient" and that the decision whether or not to operate on a patient with cirrhosis is the balance of 3 primary areas of consideration (Table 9-4): the strength of the indication of surgery, emergent and likely the patient's only hope of survival versus elective

---
Table 9-4

Patient Selection Factors in Cirrhotic Patients Being Considered for Surgery

1. Strength of surgical indication
□ Emergent potentially liver saving vs elective procedure that can be delayed or avoided
2. Risk of hepatic decompensation based on assessment of severity of current liver disease
3. Patient wishes following open discussion of factors 1 and 2

Table 9-5

Child-Turcotte-Pugh Classification of Cirrhosis

Point Value	1	2	3
Ascites	None	Mild	Moderate
Total bilirubin	< 2 mg/dL	2 to 3 mg/dL	> 3 mg/dL
Albumin	> 3.5 g/dL	2.8 to 3.5 g/dL	< 2.8 g/dL
INR	< 1.7	1.7 to 2.3	> 2.3
Encephalopathy	None	Grade 1 to 2	Grade 3 to 4
Classification	**Score**	**Estimated 90-Day Postoperative Mortality (%)**	
• Child's A	5 to 6 points	10	
• Child's B	7 to 9 points	30	
• Child's C	10 to 15 points	90	
INR indicates international normalized ratio			

procedures that can safely be delayed or avoided. A second factor is the risk of hepatic decompensation associated with the patient's existing liver disease; defining this aspect of the equation is the focus of the remaining sections of this chapter. Finally, what are the patient's wishes regarding the operation? In order for the patient to make an educated and informed choice regarding his or her options, care must be taken to determine as accurately as possible the risks of the operation, including assessment of experience and expertise of the team performing the procedure and postoperative patient management.

A number of models to predict the risk of morbidity and mortality in surgical patients with cirrhosis have been described. The most commonly utilized models will be discussed, including the American Society of Anesthesiologists physical status class (ASA class),[26] Child-Turcotte-Pugh (CTP) classification (Table 9-5),[27] and the model for end-stage liver disease (MELD) score (Table 9-6).[28]

Table 9-6

Model for End-Stage Liver Disease Score

Revised MELD formula = 3.8(ln serum bilirubin mg/dL) + 11.2(ln INR) + 9.6(serum creatinine mg/dL) + 6.4	
MELD < 10	Low surgical risk of mortality
MELD 10 to 15	Moderate surgical risk of mortality
MELD > 15	High surgical risk of mortality
MELD indicates model for end-stage liver disease; INR, international normalized ratio	

Until recently, the duration of increased risk had not been well described; however, a retrospective study by Teh et al[29] of 772 cirrhotic patients undergoing major digestive, orthopedic, or cardiovascular surgery over a period of 24 years identified an increased risk of mortality that was present during the first 90 days postoperatively compared to controls. Mortality was not different among groups at 1 year and beyond. This risk was independent of both age and MELD score. This study also found that an ASA class V preoperatively was the strongest predictor of mortality during the first 7 days postoperatively. This increased mortality may reflect cardiopulmonary rather than hepatic morbidity. It is worth noting that even patients with well-compensated cirrhosis minimally meet ASA class III requirements.

The CTP model was originally designed to predict mortality following portacaval shunt surgery[27] and was the first model used to predict surgical risk in patients with underlying liver disease. The CTP score is derived from 5 clinical variables (see Table 9-5). Patients receive 1 to 3 points for each variable and the total score, between 5 and 15, is used to determine the CTP class: A, B, or C. The CTP score has been widely used for a number of years to predict mortality in cirrhotic patients undergoing surgery, and this use is based on the results of 2 retrospective studies of approximately 100 cirrhotic patients each that identified the CTP class as the best predictor of postoperative mortality and morbidity. Both groups found mortality at 90 days of 10%, 30%, and 80% in CTP class A, B, and C patients, respectively.[7,30]

The partially subjective nature of the degree of hepatic encephalopathy and ascites inherent to the CTP model has resulted in the identification of a need to develop a more accurate method of risk assessment in patients with liver disease. The MELD score (see Table 9-6) was developed to predict short-term mortality in cirrhotic patients undergoing transjugular intrahepatic portosystemic shunt (TIPS) procedures.[31] The MELD score is a logarithmic formula based on 3 variables that produces a score from 6 to 40, with higher values indicating progressively worsening liver disease. Since 2002 the MELD score has been utilized in the United States to allocate organs to liver transplant patients to give priority to the sickest patients with the highest risk of pretransplant mortality.[32]

A number of studies have retrospectively examined the ability of the MELD score to predict perioperative mortality in patients undergoing a variety of cardiac, orthopedic, and abdominal procedures, including hepatic resection in both emergent and elective settings.[33-36] The study by Teh et al[29] found that for MELD scores < 8 the 30-day mortality was 6% and increased to 90% with a MELD score > 25. Additionally, each 1-point increase in MELD above 8 corresponded with a 14% increase in 30-day mortality. General recommendations regarding surgical candidacy for elective procedures have been proposed by Hanje and Patel.[8] Patients with MELD scores < 10 may proceed with surgery, whereas surgery should be avoided in patients with MELD scores > 15. Consideration should be given to evaluation for liver transplantation in this population as appropriate. Caution is advised when considering surgery in patients with MELD scores between 10 and 15 due to increasing risk of postoperative hepatic decompensation. A recent retrospective analysis of 100 patients with cirrhosis undergoing abdominal surgery examined the role of serum albumin levels in predicting postoperative mortality at 30 days.[37] In patients with MELD scores ≥ 15 and serum albumin of ≤ 2.5 mg/dL, the 30-day mortality was 60% compared with 14% in patients with MELD scores ≥ 15 and serum albumin of ≥ 2.5 mg/dL. Thus, the addition of serum albumin appears to be of predictive value in these patients (Figure 9-1).

PERIOPERATIVE MANAGEMENT

Common complications of cirrhosis including hepatic encephalopathy, coagulopathy, renal dysfunction, malnutrition, and ascites are frequently exacerbated during the perioperative period. Anticipation and careful management to avoid and reverse these conditions may improve outcomes and reduce mortality (Table 9-7).

Physiologic stresses related to surgery, unfamiliar surroundings, narcotic analgesics, and other centrally acting medications can all lead to increased risk of hepatic encephalopathy in the perioperative patient with cirrhosis. The use of narcotic analgesics and other centrally acting medications should be kept at a minimum. Administration of oral lactulose titrated to 2 to 3 soft bowel movements daily improves symptoms compared to placebo.[38] Lactulose therapy is commonly used as the initial treatment of hepatic encephalopathy in patients with cirrhosis. Early initiation of therapy with consideration of prophylactic use in high-risk patients combined with avoidance of precipitating medications is the key to successful management. Care must also be taken to continue lactulose dosing during transitions between inpatient and outpatient settings. Oral rifaximin administered twice a day may be added for patients with encephalopathy that is refractory to lactulose or may be substituted in patients who are intolerant of lactulose therapy.

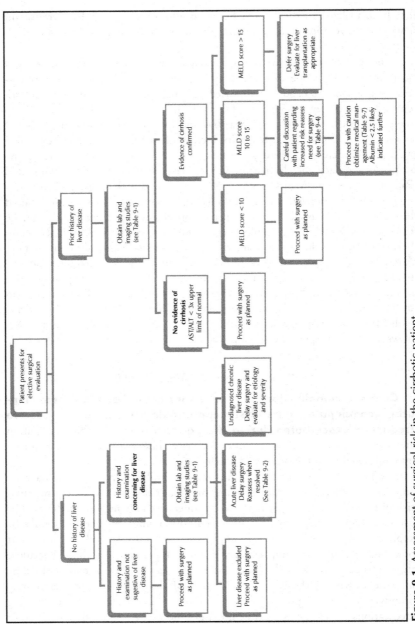

Figure 9-1. Assessment of surgical risk in the cirrhotic patient.

Table 9-7

Management Issues Requiring Special Consideration Perioperatively in Cirrhotic Patients

Potential Pitfalls	Management

■ Ascites	■ Limit crystalloid fluids
	  □ IV albumin as maintenance fluid
	■ Low-sodium diet
	■ Diuretics
	  □ Furosemide and spironolactone
	■ Large-volume paracentesis

■ Coagulopathy
  □ Target INR < 1.5
  □ Target platelets > 50,000 mm^3
	■ Vitamin K replacement
	■ Fresh-frozen plasma transfusion
	■ Platelet transfusion

■ Hepatic encephalopathy	■ Minimize use of narcotic analgesics and other central acting drugs including benzodiazepines
	■ Lactulose/rifaximin
	  □ Consider prophylactic use
	  □ Careful patient and provider instruction during transitions between inpatient and outpatient settings

■ Nutrition	■ Daily multivitamin
	  □ Zinc replacement
	■ Diet
	  □ High calorie
	  □ Low sodium
	  □ Low fat
	  □ Adequate protein

■ Renal dysfunction	■ Avoid nephrotoxic medications
	  □ Nonsteroidal anti-inflammatories
	  □ Aminoglycosides
	  □ Contrast dye
	■ Large-volume paracentesis
	  □ Replace albumin

■ Wound healing and infection	■ Excellent wound care
	  □ Careful antiseptic technique
	  □ Vigilant monitoring for infection
	  □ Antibiotics as appropriate

IV indicates intravenous; INR, international normalized ratio

Coagulopathy in patients with cirrhosis is common and may be the result of a combination of factors, including impaired synthesis of clotting factors, cholestasis, and nutritional status.[39] Administration of subcutaneous vitamin K may be helpful in reversing nutritional coagulopathy, but fresh-frozen plasma and platelet administration may be required in patients with synthetic dysfunction and significant thrombocytopenia related to splenic sequestration related to cirrhosis. A platelet count of 50,000 mm³ and an INR of < 1.5 are commonly used target levels.[12] Careful attention should also be given to optimal surgical technique; Telem et al found that operative blood loss of > 150 mL and intraoperative transfusion of packed red blood cells were strong predictors of adverse outcome in cirrhotic patients undergoing abdominal surgery.[37]

Perioperative renal dysfunction may result from decreased intravascular volume, nephrotoxic medications, and hepatorenal syndrome. **The use of potentially nephrotoxic medications such as nonsteriodal anti-inflammatories, aminoglycosides, and intravenous contrast dye should be avoided.** Patients who require large-volume paracentesis to control ascites should receive albumin infusion to avoid fluid shifts that may result in decreased renal perfusion.[40]

Patients with liver disease may have or are at risk of developing poor nutritional status. When present in patients with cirrhosis, nutritional deficiencies have a negative effect on prognosis in general and following surgery.[41,42] In addition to a multivitamin daily without iron, cirrhotic patients should follow a high-calorie, low-fat, low-sodium diet of < 2000 mg/24 h with adequate protein intake of 1.5 g/kg/day during the perioperative period.[8]

The reaccumulation of ascites postoperatively is a common problem that can lead to complications of abdominal wall hernia, wound dehiscence, spontaneous bacterial peritonitis, and compromised respiration. Efforts to prevent and control ascites must be taken, including a low-sodium diet, avoiding fluid overload by limiting crystalloid fluids, and replacing with intravenous albumin for fluid maintenance combined with appropriate use of diuretics, typically combinations of furosemide and spironolactone. Large-volume paracentesis may be used as needed for relief of tense ascites provided that appropriate albumin is given to protect renal function and to assist in increasing oncotic pressure to reduce reaccumulation.

In addition, cirrhotic patients have an increased risk of poor wound healing and infection. Therefore, excellent wound care, antiseptic techniques during wound healing, and careful monitoring for infections are of paramount importance.

CONCLUSION

Cirrhosis is a commonly encountered problem in clinical practice that is increasing in prevalence. The need for surgery in patients with cirrhosis is not uncommon, with approximately 10% of patients undergoing a surgical procedure during the last 2 years of life. Surgery in the patient with cirrhosis carries increased morbidity and mortality related to hepatic decompensation that increases with the severity of the underlying liver disease and remains present for up to 90 days postoperatively. Predictive models of perioperative morbidity and mortality including the CTP class and MELD score are available for use in stratifying patients for elective surgical procedures and may also be helpful to guide discussions with patients regarding risks and clarifying their wishes. After the decision to proceed with surgery is made, careful attention should be given to optimizing medical management of common complications of cirrhosis to reduce the risk of postoperative decompensation.

REFERENCES

1. Spraycar M, ed. *Stedman's Medical Dictionary*. 26th ed. Baltimore, MD: Williams & Wilkins; 1995.
2. Lim YS, Kim WR. The global impact of hepatic fibrosis and end-stage liver disease. *Clin Liver Dis.* 2008;12:vii, 733-746.
3. Falagas ME, Vardakas KZ, Vergidis PI. Under-diagnosis of common chronic diseases: prevalence and impact on human health. *Int J Clin Pract.* 2007;61:1569-1579.
4. Manos MM, Leyden WA, Murphy RC, Terrault NA, Bell BP. Limitations of conventionally derived chronic liver disease mortality rates: results of a comprehensive assessment. *Hepatology.* 2008;47:1150-1157.
5. Kim WR, Brown RS Jr, Terrault NA, El-Serag H. Burden of liver disease in the United States: summary of a workshop. *Hepatology.* 2002;36:227-242.
6. Schuppan D, Afdhal NH. Liver cirrhosis. *Lancet.* 2008;371:838-851.
7. Garrison RN, Cryer HM, Howard DA, Polk HC Jr. Clarification of risk factors for abdominal operations in patients with hepatic cirrhosis. *Ann Surg.* 1984;199:648-655.
8. Hanje AJ, Patel T. Preoperative evaluation of patients with liver disease. *Nat Clin Pract Gastroenterol Hepatol.* 2007;4:266-276.
9. Friedman LS. The risk of surgery in patients with liver disease. *Hepatology.* 1999;29:1617-1623.
10. Higashi H, Matsumata T, Adachi E, Taketomi A, Kashiwagi S, Sugimachi K. Influence of viral hepatitis status on operative morbidity and mortality in patients with primary hepatocellular carcinoma. *Br J Surg.* 1994;81:1342-1345.
11. Runyon BA. Surgical procedures are well tolerated by patients with asymptomatic chronic hepatitis. *J Clin Gastroenterol.* 1986;8:542-544.
12. O'Leary JG, Yachimski PS, Friedman LS. Surgery in the patient with liver disease. *Clin Liver Dis.* 2009;13:211-231.
13. Sato K, Kawamura T, Wakusawa R. Hepatic blood flow and function in elderly patients undergoing laparoscopic cholecystectomy. *Anesth Analg.* 2000;90:1198-1202.
14. Malik SM, Ahmad J. Preoperative risk assessment for patients with liver disease. *Med Clin North Am.* 2009;93:917-929,ix.
15. Schemel WH. Unexpected hepatic dysfunction found by multiple laboratory screening. *Anesth Analg.* 1976;55:810-812.
16. Ioannou GN, Boyko EJ, Lee SP. The prevalence and predictors of elevated serum aminotransferase activity in the United States in 1999-2002. *Am J Gastroenterol.* 2006;101:76-82.
17. Ioannou GN, Weiss NS, Boyko EJ, Mozaffarian D, Lee SP. Elevated serum alanine aminotransferase activity and calculated risk of coronary heart disease in the United States. *Hepatology.* 2006;43:1145-1151.
18. Harville DD, Summerskill WH. Surgery in acute hepatitis. Causes and effects. *JAMA.* 1963;184:257-261.

19. Powell-Jackson P, Greenway B, Williams R. Adverse effects of exploratory laparotomy in patients with unsuspected liver disease. *Br J Surg.* 1982;69:449-451.

20. Greenwood SM, Leffler CT, Minkowitz S. The increased mortality rate of open liver biopsy in alcoholic hepatitis. *Surg Gynecol Obstet.* 1972;134:600-604.

21. Gholson CF, Provenza JM, Bacon BR. Hepatologic considerations in patients with parenchymal liver disease undergoing surgery. *Am J Gastroenterol.* 1990;85:487-496.

22. Ceccanti M, Attili A, Balducci G, et al. Acute alcoholic hepatitis. *J Clin Gastroenterol.* 2006;40:833-841.

23. Cheung RC, Hsieh F, Wang Y, Pollard JB. The impact of hepatitis C status on postoperative outcome. *Anesth Analg.* 2003;97:550-554.

24. Csikesz NG, Nguyen LN, Tseng JF, Shah SA. Nationwide volume and mortality after elective surgery in cirrhotic patients. *J Am Coll Surg.* 2009;208:96-103.

25. Henderson JM. What are the risks of general surgical abdominal operations in patients with cirrhosis? *Clin Gastroenterol Hepatol.* 2010;8:399-400.

26. Ziser A, Plevak DJ, Wiesner RH, Rakela J, Offord KP, Brown DL. Morbidity and mortality in cirrhotic patients undergoing anesthesia and surgery. *Anesthesiology.* 1999;90:42-53.

27. Child CG, Turcotte JG. Surgery and portal hypertension. *Major Probl Clin Surg.* 1964;1:1-85.

28. Kamath PS, Wiesner RH, Malinchoc M, et al. A model to predict survival in patients with end-stage liver disease. *Hepatology.* 2001;33:464-470.

29. Teh SH, Nagorney DM, Stevens SR, et al. Risk factors for mortality after surgery in patients with cirrhosis. *Gastroenterology.* 2007;132:1261-1269.

30. Mansour A, Watson W, Shayani V, Pickleman J. Abdominal operations in patients with cirrhosis: still a major surgical challenge. *Surgery.* 1997;122:730-735;discussion 5-6.

31. Malinchoc M, Kamath PS, Gordon FD, et al. A model to predict poor survival in patients undergoing transjugular intrahepatic portosystemic shunts. *Hepatology.* 2000;31:864-871.

32. Wiesner R, Edwards E, Freeman R, et al. Model for end-stage liver disease (MELD) and allocation of donor livers. *Gastroenterology.* 2003;124:91-96.

33. Farnsworth N, Fagan SP, Berger DH, Awad SS. Child-Turcotte-Pugh versus MELD score as a predictor of outcome after elective and emergent surgery in cirrhotic patients. *Am J Surg.* 2004;188:580-583.

34. Befeler AS, Palmer DE, Hoffman M, Longo W, Solomon H, Di Bisceglie AM. The safety of intra-abdominal surgery in patients with cirrhosis: model for end-stage liver disease score is superior to Child-Turcotte-Pugh classification in predicting outcome. *Arch Surg.* 2005;140: 650-654;discussion 5.

35. Suman A, Barnes DS, Zein NN, Levinthal GN, Connor JT, Carey WD. Predicting outcome after cardiac surgery in patients with cirrhosis: a comparison of Child-Pugh and MELD scores. *Clin Gastroenterol Hepatol.* 2004;2:719-723.

36. Cucchetti A, Ercolani G, Vivarelli M, et al. Impact of model for end-stage liver disease (MELD) score on prognosis after hepatectomy for hepatocellular carcinoma on cirrhosis. *Liver Transpl.* 2006;12:966-971.

37. Telem DA, Schiano T, Goldstone R, et al. Factors that predict outcome of abdominal operations in patients with advanced cirrhosis. *Clin Gastroenterol Hepatol.* 8:451-457,quiz e58.

38. Als-Nielsen B, Gluud LL, Gluud C. Non-absorbable disaccharides for hepatic encephalopathy: systematic review of randomised trials. *BMJ.* 2004;328:1046.

39. French CJ, Bellomo R, Angus P. Cryoprecipitate for the correction of coagulopathy associated with liver disease. *Anaesth Intensive Care.* 2003;31:357-361.

40. Moreau R, Lebrec D. Diagnosis and treatment of acute renal failure in patients with cirrhosis. *Best Pract Res Clin Gastroenterol.* 2007;21:111-123.

41. Tsiaousi ET, Hatzitolios AI, Trygonis SK, Savopoulos CG. Malnutrition in end stage liver disease: recommendations and nutritional support. *J Gastroenterol Hepatol.* 2008;23:527-533.

42. Merli M, Nicolini G, Angeloni S, Riggio O. Malnutrition is a risk factor in cirrhotic patients undergoing surgery. *Nutrition.* 2002;18:978-986.

chapter

TIMING OF REFERRAL
FOR LIVER TRANSPLANT

James R. Burton, Jr, MD

Due to the success of liver transplantation over the past 2 decades, patients with end-stage liver disease have potential for improved survival and quality of life. With this advance, the gap between organ availability and demand has widened. Currently there are nearly 16,000 patients awaiting liver transplantation in the United States with about 6000 liver transplants annually and approximately 2000 deaths occurring while on the waiting list. The main indication for liver transplantation in the United States is complications of end-stage liver disease from hepatitis C virus (HCV) with or without a contributing factor of alcohol abuse. According to recent Scientific Registry of Transplant Recipients (SRTR) data, adjusted 1-year and 5-year survival after liver transplantation is 87% and 73%, respectively.

HISTORY OF LIVER ALLOCATION
IN THE UNITED STATES

The world's first liver transplant was performed by Dr. Thomas Starzl in 1963; the first *successful* transplant was performed in 1967. In 1983, a National Institutes of Health consensus conference affirmed that liver transplantation was no longer experimental and it was deemed a therapeutic modality to manage end-stage liver disease. By 1987 the demand for organs quickly surpassed supply. **At that time organ allocation was based on a policy of "sickest first" determined by the Child-Turcotte-Pugh (CTP) score, which**

Zaman A. *Managing the Complications
of Cirrhosis: A Practical Approach* (pp 125-136).
© 2012 Taylor & Francis Group.

Table 10-1

Child-Turcotte-Pugh Scoring System

Clinical or Biochemical Measurement	Points†		
	1	2	3
Hepatic encephalopathy	None	I to II	III to IV
Ascites	None	Mild	Moderate
Total bilirubin (mg/dL)	< 2.0	2.0 to 3.0	> 3.0
Serum albumin (g/dL)	> 3.5	2.8 to 3.5	< 2.8
INR	< 1.7	1.7 to 2.3	> 2.3

INR indicates international normalized ratio
†Class A = 5 to 6 points, Class B = 7 to 9 points, Class C = 10 to 15 points

was developed in the mid-1960s to predict the risk of death from undergoing surgical shunt surgery for variceal bleeding (Table 10-1). In 1997, minimum listing criteria were developed (ie, CTP score ≥ 7). Though it helps to establish indications for liver transplantation, this allocation system failed to stratify a large number of patients with end-stage liver disease on the waiting list by urgency due to a limited number of statuses (2A, 2B, and 3). As a result, waiting time played a significant role as a tiebreaker, leading to an incentive to list patients as early as possible. Additionally, because the CTP score includes subjective parameters (eg, ascites and encephalopathy), there was potential for gaming of the system. Finally, this allocation system was never validated for patients on the liver transplant waiting list.

DEVELOPMENT OF THE MODEL FOR END-STAGE LIVER DISEASE SCORE

Allocation System

In 1998, the Final Rule was issued by the Department of Health and Human Resources under the National Organ Transplant Act, which mandated that (1) organs should be allocated in the order of medical urgency, (2) the role of the waiting list should be minimized, and (3) efforts should be made to avoid futile transplantation and ensure efficient use of scarce resources. At about this time, the Mayo Clinic developed a model to predict mortality in patients receiving transjugular intrahepatic portosystemic shunts (TIPS) to treat variceal bleeding or refractory ascites.[1] This model consisted of 3 objective variables (serum creatinine, serum total bilirubin, international normalized ratio [INR]) and a fourth variable based on liver disease etiology. During further evaluation,

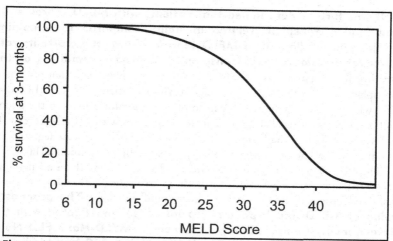

Figure 10-1. Estimated 3-month survival for patients with end-stage liver disease without liver transplant by MELD score.

etiology of liver disease was removed and a final model called the *model for end-stage liver disease* (MELD) was retrospectively and prospectively shown to be highly predictive of short-term (< 90 days) mortality in patients with all causes of end-stage liver disease, including those on the liver transplant waiting list.[2] **In February 2002, the MELD allocation system was implemented to rank patients on the liver transplant waiting list.** The MELD score used today by the United Network for Organ Sharing (UNOS) is as follows: MELD Score = $0.378 \times \log_e$ (bilirubin [mg/dL]) + $1.120 \times \log_e$ (INR) + $0.957 \times \log_e$ (creatinine [mg/dL]) + 0.643. Minimum values are set at 1.0 with a maximum creatinine of 4.0 mg/dL. For patients on dialysis 2 or more times in a prior week, creatinine level is automatically set at 4.0 mg/dL. The score ranges from 6 to 40, with 6 being normal and 40 being the highest (90% mortality at 90 days; Figure 10-1). Patients with chronic liver disease are listed on the transplant list according to blood type in rank order of MELD score from highest to lowest. A similar score was developed for pediatric patients called the *pediatric end-stage liver disease* (PELD) score, composed of bilirubin, INR, albumin, age < 1 year, and evidence of growth failure.

The impact of implementing the MELD allocation system was that compared to the era before MELD, sicker patients, as evident by higher MELD scores, were being transplanted (MELD score at transplant in pre-MELD era increased from 17 to 22 in post-MELD era) and because waiting time no longer played a significant role, the number of listings of patients with MELD scores < 10 decreased by 50%. Most important, graft and patient survival were not impacted by implementation of the MELD allocation system.

It was further determined that patients with MELD scores < 15 had higher transplant related mortality compared to remaining on the wait list (ie, only if MELD score ≥ 15 was the mortality rate lower for undergoing liver transplant compared to remaining on the waiting list).[3] This led to the Share 15 rule currently in place that prevents a transplant center from utilizing a donor organ in a patient with a MELD score < 15 without first offering the organ to other transplant centers in the region and is the basis for not listing patients for transplant with MELD scores < 15 unless the patient has had complications of end-stage liver disease (eg, variceal bleeding, ascites, hepatic encephalopathy, hepatocellular carcinoma [HCC]).

The MELD score may not accurately reflect risk of death in all patients. Hyponatremia in patients with cirrhosis is associated with refractory ascites, development of hepatorenal syndrome, and mortality. **The prognostic value of MELD and hyponatremia has been investigated with the development of a new scoring system called MELD-Na: MELD-Na = MELD − Na − (0.025 × MELD × [140 − Na]) + 140.**[4] When adjusting for MELD score, a decrease in the serum sodium concentration was associated with an increased risk of death on the waiting list. The effect of hyponatremia gradually diminishes as the MELD score increases such that the benefit of MELD-Na is seen in patients with low MELD scores. For example, a patient with a MELD score of 12 and serum sodium of 125 mmol/L would have a MELD-Na of 23 (ie, 11 points added to the MELD score), a risk of death equivalent to a MELD score of 23 with a normal serum sodium.

Patients with acute liver failure (ALF) are listed as Status 1 and have priority over all patients with chronic liver disease in each region ranked in order of listing date rather than by MELD score. Table 10-2 outlines criteria for Status 1 listing. Further comments on when to refer patients for transplant evaluation with diagnoses of ALF are discussed below.

Timing of Liver Transplant Referral

Determining the timing of liver transplantation referral depends on a number of disease-related complications in addition to the MELD score. **Early referral in patients with complications of end-stage liver disease is important so that a multidisciplinary approach can be taken to optimize management from time of referral to transplant.** One consideration is whether liver transplantation is even necessary, because there are a number of liver diseases for which there are effective management options other than liver transplantation (Table 10-3). Another consideration when determining the need for liver transplantation is an understanding of the natural history of the underlying liver disease without transplantation. For example, patients with well-compensated HCV cirrhosis (ie, no complications of liver disease) have about a 20% risk of developing liver-related complications (eg, ascites, encephalopathy, variceal bleeding) over a 10-year period. Once

Table 10-2

United Network for Organ Sharing Criteria for Status 1A Listing

1. Acute liver failure defined as the onset of hepatic encephalopathy within 8 weeks of the first symptoms of liver disease. The absence of preexisting liver disease is critical to the diagnosis. One of 3 criteria must be met to list an adult patient, who must be in the ICU with acute liver failure: (1) ventilator dependence, (2) requiring dialysis or equivalent, or (3) INR > 2.0;

or

2. Primary nonfunction of a transplanted liver within 7 days of implantation as defined by (a) or (b):

   (a) AST ≥ 3000 and one or both of the following:

       i. An INR ≥ 2.5

       ii. Acidosis, defined as having a pH ≤ 7.3 or venous pH ≤ 7.25 and/or lactate ≥ 4 mmol/L.

   (b) Anhepatic patient;

or

3. Hepatic artery thrombosis in a transplanted liver within 7 days of implantation, with evidence of severe liver injury as defined in 2(a) and 2(b) above; candidates with HAT in a transplanted liver within 14 days of implantation not meeting the above criteria will be listed at a MELD score of 40;

or

4. Acute decompensated Wilson's disease.

ICU indicates intensive care unit; INR, international normalized ratio; AST, aspartate aminotransferase; HAT, hepatic artery thrombosis; MELD, model for end-stage liver disease
Adapted from the United Network for Organ Sharing Policy 3.6, Organ Distribution: Allocation of Livers, 6/23/2009.

Table 10-3

Alternatives to Transplantation

Diagnosis	Therapy
Autoimmune hepatitis	Immunosuppression
Wilson's disease (copper overload)	Chelation therapy
Hemochromatosis (iron overload)	Phlebotomy
Decompensated chronic hepatitis B virus	Antiviral therapy
Hepatocellular carcinoma	Liver resection
HBV indicates hepatitis B virus	

■————————————————— Table 10-4 ——————————————————■

General Liver Transplant Evaluation

Hepatology Evaluation	**Laboratory Studies**
History	Etiology and severity of liver disease
Complications of liver disease	Creatinine clearance
Medications	Comorbid conditions (diabetes, iron over-
Allergies	load)
Physical examination	Previous infections (HBV, HCV, EBV,
Patient education	CMV, HIV, RPR)
Cardiopulmonary Assessment	**Abdominal Imaging**
EKG	Portal vein patency
Contrast-enhanced echo	Hepatocellular carcinoma
Dobutamine stress echo	**Psychosocial Assessment**
Pulmonary function tests	Psychiatric evaluation
CXR	Social work evaluation
	Patient education
Age-Appropriate Screening	Drug/alcohol rehab
Colonoscopy	
Mammography	**Financial Counseling**
Pap smear	**Surgical Assessment**

EKG indicates electrocardiogram; CXR, chest X-ray; HBV, hepatitis B virus; HCV, hepatitis C virus; EBV, Epstein-Barr virus; CMV, cytomegalovirus; HIV, human immunodeficiency virus; RPR, rapid plasma reagin

patients with HCV cirrhosis become decompensated, the 3-year mortality rate is approximately 50%. Additionally, rates of developing liver cancer in patients with HCV cirrhosis is estimated at 2% to 4% per year. Finally, though any complication of liver disease can justify evaluating a patient for liver transplantation, some complications are associated with significant patient mortality (eg, hepatorenal syndrome, refractory ascites, and hepatopulmonary syndrome).

GENERAL TRANSPLANT EVALUATION PROCESS

The process of evaluating patients for liver transplantation varies from center to center but largely includes the components listed in Table 10-4.[5] **Absolute contraindications to liver transplantation include metastatic cancer, severe cardiopulmonary disease, active drug and alcohol abuse, major psychiatric disease, and lack of social support.** Relative contraindications vary from center to center and include age; significant comorbid conditions such as obesity, diabetes, coronary artery disease, chronic kidney disease that may require simultaneous renal transplantation; and human immunodeficiency virus (HIV) infection. HIV infection had previously been considered a contraindication to transplantation; however, with the advent of highly active antiretroviral therapy, HIV infection with undetectable viral load and CD4 counts > 200 cells/μL can now be considered at some transplant centers with expertise in this area.

The evaluation by a transplant hepatologist largely involves determining the need for transplantation, considering alternatives to transplantation, and whether a candidate can survive the operation and immediate postoperative period as well as comply with complex management posttransplant.

The cardiopulmonary evaluation is to exclude coronary artery disease, valvular heart disease, cardiomyopathy, obstructive/restrictive lung disease, pulmonary hypertension, and hepatopulmonary syndrome. This assessment is done with electrocardiography, contrast echocardiography, dobutamine stress echocardiography, chest x-ray, and pulmonary function tests. In select patients this evaluation may also include cardiac catheterization.

Laboratory testing is done to confirm/determine the etiology and severity of liver disease, screen for comorbid conditions such as diabetes and iron overload, and evaluate for evidence of previous infection that may explain reason for needing transplantation (ie, hepatitis B virus [HBV] and HCV) or impact posttransplant care (ie, cytomegalovirus [CMV], Epstein-Barr virus [EBV], rapid plasma reagin [RPR]).

The psychosocial evaluation, which may include consultation with psychiatry, centers largely on a social work evaluation to identify social support and the need for drug and/or alcohol rehabilitation. Nearly all transplant centers in the United States require at least 6 months of abstinence from drugs and alcohol to be considered a transplant candidate. Issues of cigarette smoking and use of marijuana are center dependent and vary from complete abstinence as a requirement for listing to a recommendation of cessation.

Obesity (body mass index [BMI] > 30 kg/m^2) is a major problem in the United States with a prevalence in adults of over 30%. It is projected that cirrhosis from nonalcoholic steatohepatitis will become the leading indication for liver transplantation in the United States in the near future. A study analyzing the effect of obesity on post-liver transplant outcomes utilizing SRTR data suggested an increased patient mortality in patients with BMI > 35 kg/m^2. A criticism of this analysis was the way in which BMI was calculated by not correcting for ascites. Recent analysis from the Mayo Clinic revealed similar posttransplant outcomes between obese and non-obese patients when BMI was corrected for presence of ascites.[6] Results of this study do not imply that all obese patients can routinely be transplanted safely, because obese patients in this study represented a highly selected group. This study did demonstrate the importance of considering patients on an individual basis and not automatically excluding patients based on BMI. **Generally, a BMI < 35 kg/m^2 is desired in patients with comorbid conditions (ie, diabetes, hypertension, hyperlipidemia, coronary artery disease) and a BMI < 38 kg/m^2 in patients without comorbidities.**

Table 10-5

Diagnoses Meeting United Network for Organ Sharing Standardized Model for End-Stage Liver Disease Allocation Exceptions

Diagnosis	Criteria
Hepatopulmonary syndrome	1. Evidence of liver disease and/or portal hypertension 2. PaO_2 < 60 mm Hg on room air arterial blood gas 3. No significant clinical evidence of underlying primary pulmonary disease 4. Pulmonary vascular dilatation documented by positive contrast transthoracic contrast echocardiography
Portopulmonary hypertension	1. MPAP > 35 mmHg 2. Treatment of pulmonary artery hypertension with MPAP < 35 mm Hg and PVR < 400 dyne/s/cm^{-5} by heart catheterization
Cystic fibrosis	FEV_1 that falls below 40%
Familial amyloid polyneuropathy	1. Echocardiogram showing EF > 40% 2. Ambulatory status 3. Transthyretin gene mutation (Val30Met versus non-Val30Met) and biopsy-proven amyloid in the involved organ
Primary hyperoxaluria (and/or genetic analysis)	1. AGT deficiency proven by liver biopsy (sample analysis) 2. GFR ≤ 25 mL/min for at least 6 weeks 3. Listed for combined liver-kidney transplant
Cholangiocarcinoma	See Table 10-7
Hepatocellular carcinoma	See Table 10-8

MELD indicates model for end-stage liver disease; PaO2, partial pressure of oxygen in arterial blood; MPAP, mean pulmonary artery pressure; PVR, pulmonary vascular resistance; FEV_1, forced expiratory volume in the first second; EF, ejection fraction; AGT, alanine:glyoxylate aminotranferase; GFR, glomerular filtration rate
Adapted from United Network for Organ Sharing Policy 3.6, Organ Distribution: Allocation of Livers, 6/23/2009.

STANDARDIZED EXCEPTIONS FOR LIVER TRANSPLANTATION

There are a number of conditions for which the need for liver transplantation is not accurately defined by the MELD score because prognosis depends on factors other than liver-related mortality. Tables 10-5 through 10-7 outline these exceptional diagnoses. HCC is one such example, because the MELD

Table 10-6

Criteria for Standardized Model for End-Stage Liver Disease Exception for Cholangiocarcinoma

Eligible candidates:
1. Unresectable hilar cholangiocarcinoma or hilar cholangiocarcinoma in setting of primary sclerosing cholangitis
2. No clinical evidence of intrahepatic or extrahepatic metastases
3. If cross-sectional imaging demonstrates mass, the mass should be ≤ 3 cm

Diagnostic criteria:
1. Intraluminal brush cytology or biopsy
2. In case of negative cytology, malignant-appearing stricture with at least one of the following:
   (a) CA 19-9 level > 100 ng/mL
   (b) Biliary aneuploidy by DIA and/or FISH

All candidates must complete neoadjuvant therapy (radiation and chemotherapy) and undergo exploratory laparotomy prior to transplant to exclude regional hepatic lymph node involvement and peritoneal metastases.

CA 19-9 indicates carbohydrate antigen 19-9; DIA, digital image analysis; FISH, fluorescense in-situ hybridization

Adapted from the United Network for Organ Sharing Policy 3.6, Organ Distribution: Allocation of Livers, 6/23/2009.

Table 10-7

Criteria for Standardized Model for End-Stage Liver Disease Exception for Hepatocellular Carcinoma

1. Single tumor ≥ 2 cm and < 5 cm or no more than 3 lesions, with the largest < 3 cm (Milan criteria).
2. Absence of macroscopic vascular invasion and CT chest excluding metastatic disease.
3. Cross-sectional imaging should document vascular blush, an alpha-fetoprotein > 200 ng/mL, an arteriogram confirming a tumor, a biopsy confirming HCC, or chemoembolization of lesion, radiofrequency, cryo, or chemical ablation of the lesion.
4. Patient is not a candidate for resection.

CT indicates computed tomography; HCC, hepatocellular carcinoma

Adapted from United Network for Organ Sharing Policy 3.6, Organ Distribution: Allocation of Livers, 6/23/2009.

score does not reflect the risk of death or being removed from the transplant list due to tumor progression. In the case of HCC, when the MELD allocation system went into effect, estimates of probabilities of death or being removed from the transplant list were arbitrarily assigned. **The minimum criterion for priority was that HCC fall within the Milan criteria (see Table 10-7), a stage at which excellent posttransplant results had already been well established.[7] Potential recipients with HCC within the Milan criteria can receive an automatic MELD exception (22 points, with 3 additional points every 3 months until transplanted as long as candidates fulfill criteria outlined in Table 10-7).** Expansion of the UNOS criteria for transplanting HCC while maintaining similar outcomes has been undertaken by a number of groups. **One such group is the University of California– San Francisco (UCSF) and their so-called UCSF criteria.** These criteria expand a single lesion from 5 cm to 6.5 cm and for 2 to 3 tumors up to total tumor diameter of ≤ 8 cm. The group at UCSF has also reported similarly good outcomes with downstaging of tumors exceeding Milan criteria. If locoregional therapy (eg, chemoembolization, radiofrequency ablation) can lead to complete tumor necrosis such that a patient meets Milan criteria, acceptable outcomes can be expected with transplantation if the tumors remain within Milan criteria for at least 3 months. **Patients who do not meet an automatic UNOS exception for HCC but meet UCSF criteria or are downstaged into Milan can arguably request a MELD exception with the Regional Review Board.** Additionally, any individual case regardless of indication for transplantation can be appealed to the Regional Review Board for upgrade on a case-by-case basis if the transplant center feels that the risk of dying or being removed from the wait list is not reflected by a patient's MELD score.

Acute Liver Failure

ALF is a rare condition, with about 2000 cases in the United States annually.[8] It is characterized by rapid deterioration in liver function and in severe cases is associated with high mortality without liver transplantation. **The most widely accepted definition of ALF is coagulopathy (INR > 1.5), with encephalopathy occurring as the consequence of severe liver damage in patients without preexisting liver disease (exceptions include Wilson's disease, hepatitis B infection, and autoimmune hepatitis).** The leading etiologies of ALF in the United States include acetaminophen (nearly 50% of cases), drug toxicity, hepatitis B, autoimmune hepatitis, and unknown causes (10% to 20%). Diagnosis involves careful history for viral risk factors (hepatitis A virus [HAV], HBV, herpes simplex virus [HSV]), drugs (acetaminophen, antibiotics), toxins, and excluding risk factors for chronic liver disease (HCV, alcohol). **Early management of ALF involves intensive care unit (ICU) management for frequent monitoring and early communication with a transplant center.** Careful evaluation for etiology

Table 10-8

King's College Criteria for Poor Prognosis in Acute Liver Failure

Acetaminophen-Induced ALF

Arterial pH < 7.3 (after resuscitation) irrespective of coma grade

or

INR > 6.5 and serum creatinine > 3.4 in patients with grade III/IV coma

Non-Acetaminophen-Induced ALF

INR > 6.5 irrespective of degree of encephalopathy

or

Any 3 of the following, irrespective of degree of encephalopathy:

- Drug toxicity, indeterminate cause of ALF
- Age < 10 years or > 40 years
- Jaundice to coma interval > 7 days
- INR ≥ 3.5
- Serum bilirubin > 17.5 mg/dL

ALF indicates acute liver failure; INR, international normalized ratio

provides the best indicator for prognosis and may dictate a specific management (ie, N-acetylcystein for acetaminophen toxicity, steroids for autoimmune hepatitis, TIPS for acute Budd-Chiari syndrome).

The most widely accepted prognostic criteria in ALF are the King's College Criteria (Table 10-8).[9] Positive predictive values for death in the acetaminophen and non-actetominophen groups were 84% and 98%, respectively, whereas negative predictive values were 86% and 82%, respectively. Patients fulfilling these criteria have a poor prognosis for spontaneous survival and warrant urgent liver transplantation evaluation.

LIVING DONOR LIVER TRANSPLANTATION

Widely accepted for pediatric transplantation, adult-to-adult living donor liver transplantation (LDLT) is an attractive option to expand the donor pool. This technically complex operation requires a major (50% to 60%) resection of the right lobe in a healthy person to obtain an adequate graft for the recipient. Not only does LDLT avoid the waiting period for a deceased donor, it greatly reduces the ischemic period of the transplanted organ and changes the operation from an emergency into a scheduled procedure. The obvious disadvantage is that it requires placing a healthy person potentially at risk and provides the donor with a smaller portion of liver than would be received with a deceased donor graft. **In general, to be a candidate for LDLT, recipients must be candidates**

for deceased donor transplantation and have liver disease or complications of liver disease severe enough to warrant the risk of liver transplantation and potential risk to the donor. Donor qualifications and evaluations vary from center to center, but generally potential donors must have compatible blood type, be roughly the same physical size as the recipient, and be healthy without any significant medical problems.

CONCLUSION

Liver transplantation referral requires careful consideration of many issues, such as alternatives to liver transplantation, the natural history of liver disease without transplantation, the MELD score, and complications of liver disease associated with increased mortality. Successful management of these complicated patients requires a multidisciplinary approach to optimize management before transplant. **When in doubt about a patient's candidacy or indication for transplantation, make a referral or speak directly with a transplant center.**

REFERENCES

1. Malinchoc M, Kamath PS, Gordon FD, Peine CJ, Rank J, ter Borg PC. A model to predict poor survival in patients undergoing transjugular intrahepatic portosystemic shunts. *Hepatology.* 2000;31:864-871.
2. Kamath PS, Wiesner RH, Malinchoc M, et al. A model to predict surivial in patients with end-stage liver disease. *Hepatology.* 2001;33:464-470.
3. Merion RM, Schaubel DE, Kykstra DM, Freeman RB, Port FK, Wolfe RA. The survival benefit of liver transplantation. *Am J Transplant.* 2005;5:307-313.
4. Kim WR, Biggins SW, Kremers WK, et al. Hyponatremia and mortality among patients on the liver-transplant waiting list. *N Engl J Med.* 2008;359:1018-1026.
5. Murray KF, Carithers RL Jr; American Association for the Study of Liver Diseases. AASLD practice guidelines: evaluation of the patient for liver transplantation. *Hepatology.* 2005;41: 1407-1432.
6. Leonard J, Heimbach JK, Malinchoc M, et al. The impact of obesity on long-term outcomes in liver transplant recipients—results of the NIDDK liver transplant database. *Am J Transpl.* 2008;8:667-672.
7. Mazzaferro V, Regalia E, Coci R, et al. Liver transplantation for the treatment of small hepatocellular carcinomas in patients with cirrhosis. *N Engl J Med.* 1996;334:693-699.
8. Polson J, Lee WM; American Association for the Study of Liver Diseases. AASLD position paper: the management of acute liver failure. *Hepatology.* 2005;41:1179-1197.
9. O'Grady JG, Alexander GJM, Hayllar KM, Williams R. Early indictors of prognosis in fulminant hepatic failure. *Gastroenterology.* 1989;97:439-445.

FINANCIAL DISCLOSURES

James R. Burton Jr has no financial or proprietary interest in the materials presented herein.

Michael F. Chang has no financial or proprietary interest in the materials presented herein.

Jonathan M. Fenkel has no financial or proprietary interest in the materials presented herein.

Edoardo G. Giannini has no financial or proprietary interest in the materials presented herein.

Kenneth Ingram has not disclosed any relevant financial relationships

Willscott E. Naugler has no financial or proprietary interest in the materials presented herein.

Victor J. Navarro has not disclosed any relevant financial relationships

Anna Sasaki has no financial or proprietary interest in the materials presented herein.

Jonathan M. Schwartz has no financial or proprietary interest in the materials presented herein.

Jayant A. Talwalkar has no financial or proprietary interest in the materials presented herein.

Atif Zaman has no financial or proprietary interest in the materials presented herein.

INDEX

Printed in the United States
by Baker & Taylor Publisher Services